Dementia Action Plan

This book contains information about memory and brain health. This information is not intended to replace the advice, diagnosis or treatment of your doctor or other health care provider. This information is not for diagnosis or treatment of any physical or emotional condition. It is recommended that you seek your physician's advice before using the information in this book. The publisher and author disclaims liability for any adverse effects or medical outcomes as a result of applying the information presented herein.

Names: Sagha, Hamid Reza, 1968- author.

Title: Dementia action plan : give your brain a fighting chance! / Hamid Reza Sagha, MD.

Description: Forsyth, IL : Interact Well Care, 2019.

Identifiers: LCCN 2019911079 (print) | ISBN 978-1-73371-610-9 (paperback) | ISBN 978-1-73371-612-3 (Kindle ebook) | ISBN 978-1-73371-611-6 (epub ebook)

Subjects: LCSH: Dementia. | Dementia--Prevention. | Alzheimer's disease. | Cognition--Age factors. | Aging. | Health. | BISAC: HEALTH & FITNESS / Diseases / Alzheimer's & Dementia. | HEALTH & FITNESS / Healthy Living.

Classification: LCC RC521 .S23 2019 (print) | LCC RC521 (ebook) | DDC 616.8/3--dc23.

Printed in the United States of America
Library of Congress Control Number: 2019911079
First Printing, 2019
ISBN 9781733716109

Interact Well Care
332 W Marion Ave., Suite S1
Forsyth, IL 62535
www.interactwellcare.com

Dementia Action Plan

Give Your Brain a Fighting Chance!

WRITTEN BY: HAMID REZA SAGHA, M.D.

FOREWORD BY: TERRY WAHLS, M.D.

To my father, Hassan, and all other seniors on Earth.

Table of Contents

Foreword

by Dr. Terry Wahls, MD

Clinical Professor of Medicine
University of Iowa College of Medicine

If you wish to limit your risk of Alzheimer's and other dementias, *Dementia Action Plan*, by Hamid Sagha, will provide you with the knowledge and skills to do so. By implementing his suggestions for better lifestyle choices, you will both reduce your chances of getting Alzheimer's and improve your overall health.

Alzheimer's dementia is a complex disease, but you won't have trouble understanding this book. Hamid presents his information in an accessible and easy-to-digest fashion. He's also careful to avoid promises that our current understanding of dementia cannot support. There's no talk of curing Alzheimer's or reversing its effects. Instead, he explains the risk factors that you can address so that you can enhance the ability of your body's organs and systems to resist memory loss.

He has made similar lifestyle changes in his own life and freely admits that the changes were difficult. Because of his own experience, he does not expect you to rely on willpower alone to make these changes. Instead, he includes an honest discussion of how to form new, robust routines and habits that will enable you to take control of your health—skillpower, he says, rather than willpower.

He understands that we each have our own unique drive, limitations and abilities. After providing the building blocks of knowledge and understanding, he encourages us to create our own personalized plan for reducing our risk of dementia, one that reflects the healthy habits we already have and the changes we need to make for even better health.

As you read the book, you will see very quickly that Hamid is on your side. He wants you to succeed. More than that, he believes you will succeed. He genuinely wants the years ahead of you to be richer in energy, comfort and vitality, and his faith in your ability to improve your health and your body's desire to thrive is both inspiring and empowering.

Dementia Action Plan offers you a chance to fight for your life and your memories—and win!

Preface

My Journey to Better Health

> *"The knowledge of anything, since all things have causes, is not acquired or complete unless known by causes. Therefore, in medicine we ought to know the causes of sickness and health."*
>
> — *Avicenna, Prince of Physicians*

I almost died twice.

The first time was in 2007. I went into cardiac arrest, and my heart stopped beating for eight seconds.

I was working as a doctor at a hospital at the time. Instead of putting myself under a cardiologist's care, I decided to treat myself. I knew what to do. I was certain disease care would solve my problems, so I took cholesterol and blood pressure medications and went on with my life.

But I never dealt with the underlying causes of my heart disease. I kept drinking too many soft drinks, smoking, gaining weight and never exercising, so I became sicker and sicker.

I remember going to New York City with my family to watch the ball drop at Times Square on New Year's Eve. We did a little sightseeing, ate delicious food, and by the time evening came, I didn't have the energy or the desire to go with my family to Times Square.

I have a picture from that trip. I looked close to death. And I was—closer than I realized.

My second wake-up call came in 2013, a few months after my trip to New York City. Alone in a hotel room, preparing to go to one of my out-of-town jobs as a doctor, I went to get a drink of water and woke up on the floor. I had passed out and was bleeding from a cut on my forehead. I somehow managed to drag myself to my phone to call 911.

At that time of my life, I was working long hours in an emergency room, smoking, eating way too much and sleeping only four or five hours each day. I drank coffee frequently but still had trouble staying awake. I was often short of breath and had to use a CPAP machine to sleep.

I was also taking three blood pressure medications every day that failed to bring my systolic pressure any lower than 190, and along with taking both Zantac and Protonix for my acid reflux, I bought Tums in bulk.

Worst of all, I had lost my ability to think clearly. I had always loved to learn and had enjoyed using that learning on behalf of my patients in the emergency room.

But now, because of brain fog, it was becoming harder and harder to stay sharp, alert and equipped to do my job.

As I lay in the hospital following my cardiac arrest, I couldn't help wondering, *What is wrong with me?*

My grandfather, who lived until he was 100, never took medication, and my father, who was 90 at the time, had never been as sick as I was.

I was a physician who had worked in two different countries. I was familiar with various health care systems, from traditional to conventional to modern medicine. I had worked for many years in many settings—a clinic, a nursing home facility, a hospital and currently in an emergency and critical care setting.

And yet there I was, in my late 40s, and I had almost died.

That second brush with death was a turning point for me. After that I began working on the causes of my poor health.

I lost 70 pounds. My triglycerides went from 480 to 80. My blood sugar level is now normal. I exercise daily without any shortness of breath. I have stopped smoking and eat a healthy, plant-based diet. At 50, I am healthier than I have ever been. Best of all, my mind is sharp again.

Through all these changes, I have been carrying out an intensive personal research project on my own body, looking beyond the symptoms to the causes of my poor health.

Lifestyle Choices and Chronic Disease

But wait! you might say. *This book is about Alzheimer's disease, not heart problems.*

You are correct, but the root causes of my illness were the lifestyle choices I was making. These included a life of constant stress, poor nutrition, lack of sleep, a sedentary lifestyle, smoking and eating way too much sugar.

When I addressed these modifiable lifestyle choices—in other words, when I got rid of the garbage in my life—my body was able to heal.

Remember my foggy thinking? I believe that was an inflammatory response to my lifestyle. I am still amazed at how much sharper my cognitive abilities are today compared to those dark days when I was so sick and didn't even realize it.

The book you are reading reflects my experience of changing my lifestyle choices. The same process can guide you in your efforts to reduce your risk of Alzheimer's dementia.

Why I Chose to Write About Dementia

Dementia describes a group of symptoms related to memory and mental reasoning. Alzheimer's dementia is the most common disease that includes this group of symptoms.

Again and again, in the ER where I work, I see patients with Alzheimer's dementia. Often the patients have reached the stage where their anxieties make them violent, and their families are seeking some medication that will calm the patients down so that they can continue to receive care at home.

For a long time, all I could do was prescribe some drug that will, at best, slow down the progression of Alzheimer's a little. After millions of dollars and decades of research, we still do not have an effective treatment for Alzheimer's dementia once the symptoms appear.

In the ER, I also saw the effect of Alzheimer's on caregivers, the unsung heroes of our society, and I deeply, passionately wanted to relieve their anxieties and burdens as well.

I became so distressed by the suffering of my patients and their caregivers that I began to wonder if addressing modifiable lifestyle changes—as I had in my own life—might also reduce the risk of Alzheimer's dementia.

So I began an in-depth study of Alzheimer's dementia, seeking ways we can all reduce our risk of developing this devastating disease. This book offers the insights and results of my study.

When patients with Alzheimer's dementia come to the ER, I still can't do much for their disease, but I can offer some hope to their caregivers about how they can reduce their risk of developing the same symptoms—especially if they are willing to start long before the symptoms might first appear.

I want to offer you that same hope and enable you to explore new and better opportunities for cognitive health. In this book, I describe a healing process based on lifestyle choices that anyone can choose for his or her own life, without expensive doctors, programs or treatment plans.

Your body wants to be healthy and vibrant. You can help your body achieve that goal. This can be your guidebook as you embark on a journey toward understanding, new habits, better choices and greater well-being.

Can Anyone Prevent Alzheimer's?

In a word: *No.*

Many scientists and health professionals are investigating Alzheimer's dementia, rapidly expanding our knowledge of this disease, but our understanding of what causes the disease is still incomplete.

So a guaranteed way to prevent Alzheimer's dementia is still in the future.

Instead, current research is identifying many associations or correlations between lifestyle choices and their potential to increase or reduce the risk of Alzheimer's dementia.

For the sake of transparency, I avoid overselling these strategies as guarantees. Instead, I want to offer you the best possible recommendations for protecting your cognitive and physical health. Transparency is also why I frequently refer to factors that contribute to Alzheimer's rather than cause it.

We hope that research into these correlations eventually leads to causal connections and guaranteed solutions to this disease.

That's how it worked with bacteria and infection. For many years, surgeons failed to recognize that dirty hands contributed to infectious diseases. Then someone saw that patients were less likely to become infected if surgeons washed their hands. In other words, someone established a correlation.

Initially, there was significant resistance to the claim that surgeons should wash their hands. *"I'm making my patients sick? No!"*

But research established a stronger and stronger causal relationship, and soon surgeons began testing the idea themselves. When they did so, incidents of infection decreased. Today, a sterile environment for surgery is standard.

Perhaps someday, some of the correlations we now see between healthy choices and Alzheimer's dementia will lead to an understanding of actual causes. In the meantime, these correlations offer practical strategies that might help you avoid Alzheimer's.

All for the Best

If you get started making step-by-step changes and keep going, you will not only improve your overall health, you will reduce your risk of dementia in general, and specifically Alzheimer's, at the same time.

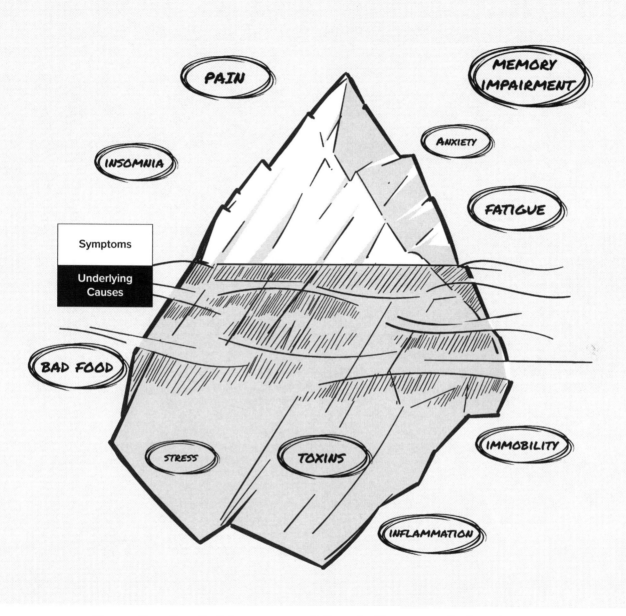

Examples of underlying causes of chronic disease, including dementia

Introduction

A Framework for Your Personalized Dementia Action Plan

A comprehensive approach to your journey.

What a Dementia Action Plan is <u>not</u>: A daily diet to follow, a bundle of supplements to take, a piece of equipment to buy, an exercise plan, a set of mind games to buy or even a prescribed sequence of steps to follow.

What it is: Your own plan—based on your own decisions and design—for changing the lifestyle choices that are putting you at risk for dementia.

I recommend five stages for you to work through as you create and fulfill your personalized plan. You will probably move up and down and around these stages, but they will provide the structure for your plan.

Stage 1: Preparation—Willpower

For this journey, you will need to step out of your comfort zone and change many of your routines. Deciding that you are ready to do this is the first, bedrock stage of any dementia plan. This means you have the initial **Willpower** to begin this journey.

I hope you are holding this book because you have already made this decision. I also hope you are starting this journey before you experience any symptoms of memory loss or cognitive decline. This is the ideal time because the damage begins before symptoms appear.

If you have already begun to experience symptoms, this is still a great time to embark on your dementia plan. There's much you can do to reduce your additional risk of dementia.

Please consider this question carefully. If you are doing this for someone else, or if you are reluctant or unwilling to change, this isn't the right time for you. Come back when you are ready!

Stage 2: Your Emotional Outlook

At every level, through all that you do, your emotional outlook is central to your success. It's the load-bearing wall of your Dementia Action Plan structure.

Like all of us, you are human. You have failed yourself and your loved ones. In your turn, you have also been wronged, often unjustly. Quite possibly those closest to you have betrayed and wounded you.

Forgiving yourself and others is of paramount importance because the ongoing anger and resentment will hurt your health, contributing to stress, high blood pressure, loss of sleep, fatigue, overeating and depression. Anger and resentment are a deadly burden on your body, mind and spirit.

When you forgive, you can mindfully seek instead to love yourself and others. This love and kindness will fortify all your efforts on this journey away from dementia and permeate your life with hope, confidence and joy.

So please don't lose sight of your emotional outlook as you pursue your personalized dementia plan. Everything else in your plan depends on this central pillar.

Stage 3: Education—Skillpower

To succeed, you'll need more than *Willpower*. You'll need the *Skillpower* which can only come from an understanding of yourself, dementia and what you can do to reduce your risk factors.

Your knowledge and understanding will be powerful weapons in your fight for cognitive health.

About yourself, ask:

Why are you doing this? Make a list, put it on your refrigerator, and add to it when new motivations come to mind. These will be very important to you.

What are your current routines and habits? What critical moments trigger these routines and what rewards do you get from each? Consider especially the routines that might harm you. Is there something you can do to make them less attractive? Is there anything you can do to make healthy habits more attractive?

What social support do you have? Is your spouse or partner on board with the changes you'll be making? Is there someone who can be your unofficial accountability partner to check up on your progress and encourage you?

What is most likely to improve your motivation? What might present obstacles?

About dementia:

You'll need to know your enemy. **Section 1** of this book, *Dementia Action Plan*, will inform you about dementia, and more particularly Alzheimer's dementia. It will explain inflammation, which is central to cognitive decline (and other chronic diseases). I also include an encouraging chapter on genes and our ability to change their expression.

Take advantage of these chapters at this stage.

About reducing your risk:

Section 2 of *Dementia Action Plan* explains modifiable lifestyle changes you can make to decrease your risk of Alzheimer's dementia.

Each chapter also offers specific action steps you can include in your personalized plan, but for this stage just acquaint yourself with the content. Specific planning will occur at the next stage, when you will be able to choose what risk factors to work on first and what action steps will make the most difference in your life.

As you read through these chapters, you may decide to make specific preparations such as a pantry intervention to remove harmful foods from your home, purchasing water and air filtration devices and other changes. (You can also choose to make these changes later as you work on your lifestyle changes.)

Section 3 explains two important elements you can add to your life: social connections and learning.

As you work on Stage 3, our website, InteractWellCare.com, has many other resources you can access, including easy-to-understand videos on many topics and tools for your preparations.

Section 4 of the book follows up with a frank discussion about the difficulties you'll encounter on your journey, and up-to-date suggestions for forming new, robust routines and habits that will reduce your risk of Alzheimer's.

Take your time with this stage. The more you know and understand, the better your chance of success. Willpower + Skillpower!

Stage 4: Modifiable Lifestyle Changes

In this book, we focus on Alzheimer's dementia because it is the most common and deadly form of dementia and because reducing your risk of

Alzheimer's dementia will help you guard against other forms of dementia as well.

There is no cure for Alzheimer's yet, but research has identified risk factors for the disease. From these, we have identified seven changes in your lifestyle that will decrease your personal risk. We call these Modifiable Lifestyle Changes.

They include:

- Improving your sleep
- Moving more (exercise)
- Eating healthy food
- Decreasing stress
- Detoxifying your air, water and environment
- Improving your social connections
- Increasing your sensory and mental stimulation

Interact Well Care is here for you as you embark on making these lifestyle changes. We have designed an integrated system starting with the *Dementia Action Plan* book. **Sections 2 and 3** provide essential information about the modifiable lifestyle changes, as well as detailed suggestions for change.

Our website, InteractWellCare.com, offers many additional resources.

Stage 5: System Health

In this stage, you will apply what you have learned about your body's systems and organs so you can have better metabolism, biology, health and well-being. Let's look at these systems one by one:

- **Your endocrine system:** In this book, you'll learn about hormones and their essential role in your cognitive health. As you apply what you learn, your hormones will become more balanced, so cells in your body can communicate better.

- **Your immune system:** The immune system is your body's friend and protector and also your body's foe—depending on whether an immune response produces acute or chronic inflammation. You'll be learning the difference between these two in this book, as well as why inflammation can become chronic. As you take steps to decrease chronic inflammation, you'll make a critical difference in your cognitive health and in any chronic diseases you may have. You'll also learn how to strengthen your immune system for the sake of your overall health.

- **Your detoxifying organs:** In this book, you will also learn about the many modifiable lifestyle choices you can make to eliminate toxins and contaminants from your air, water and environment. You'll also learn how you can strengthen the organs that detoxify your body, specifically your skin, lungs, gut, kidney, liver and lymphatic systems.

- **Your mitochondria:** Mitochondria help to supply energy to every cell in your body, so your life depends on them. You'll learn more about them in this book and about how you can protect mitochondria and optimize their function.

- **Your digestive system and gut:** Because your brain and gut are connected by an express freeway of nerves, what happens in your gut strongly influences what happens in your brain. You'll be applying what you learn about the gut and microbiome to improve the digestion and absorption of the food you eat and to protect your gut from harmful bacteria. This system is vitally important to your cognitive health.

- **Your lungs, heart and musculoskeletal system:** As you improve your lifestyle choices, your lungs will more efficiently provide oxygen to your cells and remove carbon dioxide from your body. Your heart will deliver nutrients and oxygen to cells throughout your body more effectively. Your muscles and bones will provide better support and movement for your body and fulfill their other important functions better.

The figure on the next page illustrates the dementia action plan. Learning more about how these systems *Interact* together for better *Well Care* will have a significant impact on your overall health. A new life is ahead!

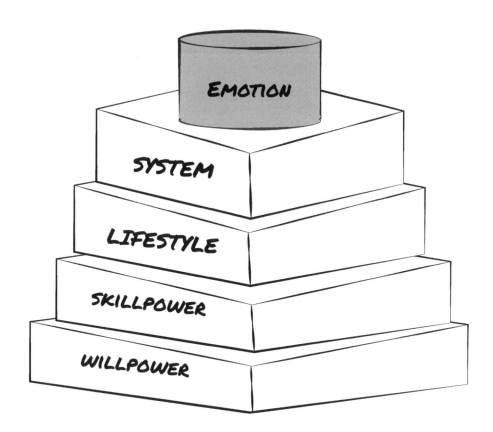

Maintenance

As I mentioned, these stages are not sequential steps. Your emotional outlook supports every stage, and as you work on your plan, you will need to move back and forth through all the stages.

You will also encounter relapses and the need to revise plans and motivations. Keep going! Eventually your new lifestyle choices will settle into routines, and it will be easier to maintain them. That's the goal.

The Best Time Is Now!

This framework will help you design your own Dementia Action Plan. It provides a comprehensive approach to your journey away from dementia to a better memory.

The best time to start is today, so you can enjoy your new brain and your new you!

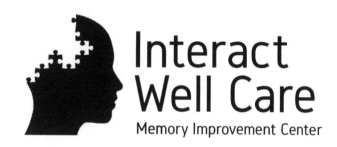

Interact
Well Care
Memory Improvement Center

InteractWellCare.com
info@InteractWellCare.com

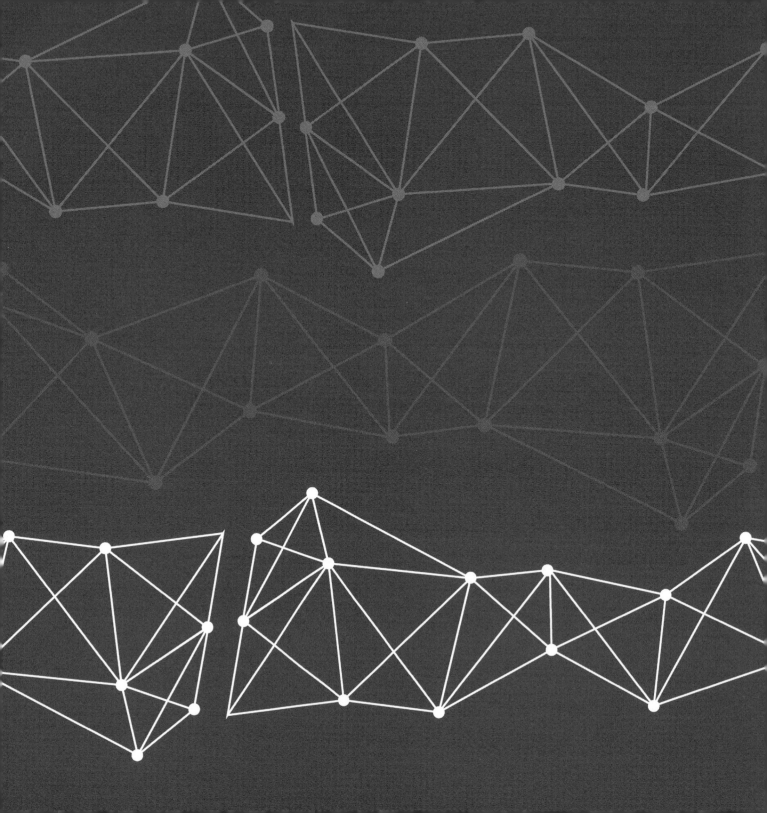

Section 1

*Definitions,
Explanations
and
Context*

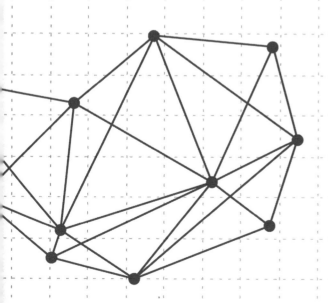

Chapter 1

Cognitive
Impairment:
What We
Should Know

The brain has billions of neurons, each capable of building new connections.

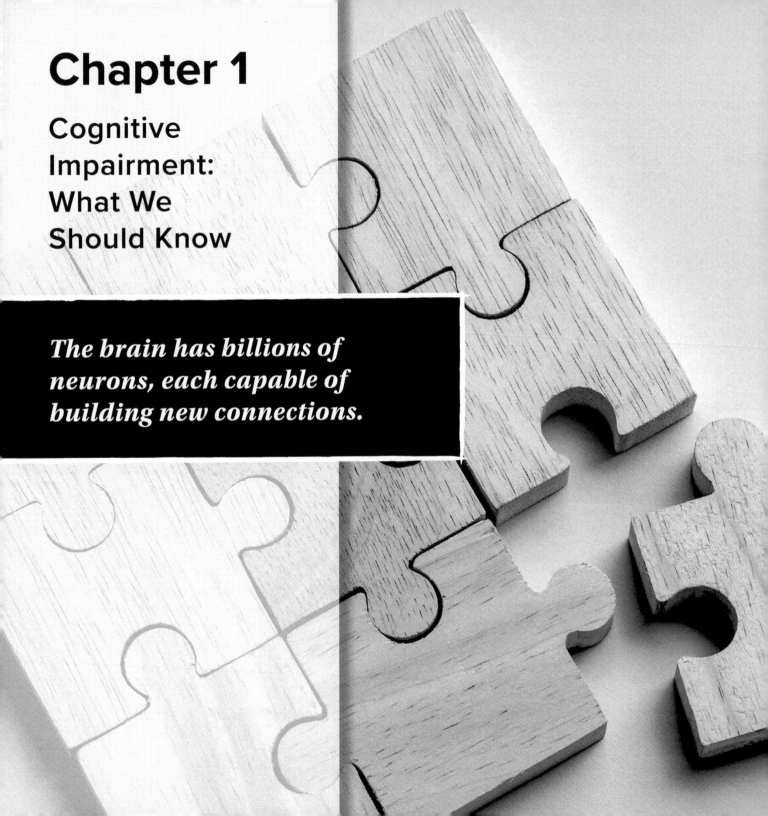

Dementia is not a disease. It is an umbrella term applied to a group of symptoms related to memory, as well as the ability to perform daily activities, make plans and communicate with others.

These dementia-related diseases include Alzheimer's dementia, vascular dementia, Lewy body dementia, Parkinson's disease and others.

Alzheimer's dementia is the most common cause of the symptoms associated with dementia. It accounts for 60% to 80% of cases,[1] and it is the sixth-leading cause of death in the United States. Every 65 seconds, doctors diagnose one of our fellow citizens with this disease.

Because it is the most common form of dementia, this book focuses primarily on Alzheimer's dementia. Bear in mind, however, that if you reduce your risk of Alzheimer's dementia, you will also be reducing your risk of dementia in general, as well as many other health problems.

Alzheimer's dementia has three hallmarks:

1. Cell death, leading to brain shrinkage
2. Beta-amyloid plaques
3. Neurofibrillary, or tau, tangles

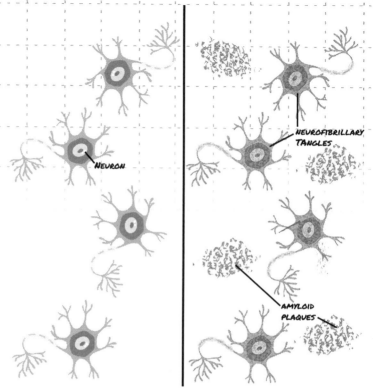

Hallmarks of dementia: plaques and tangles.

Hallmark #1: Cell Death

Symptoms of Alzheimer's dementia occur when nerve cells, or neurons, die. These deaths cause the brain to shrink. With widespread cell death, the patient's ability to reason suffers.

The nervous system includes both the central nervous system (your brain and your spinal cord) and the peripheral nervous system (the nerves that run throughout your body).[2] Your nervous system is an amazingly powerful chemical and electrical complex. It lets you see, hear, touch, talk, move, feel—and most importantly for dementia—remember and make decisions.

The nervous system has more than 100 billion neurons that carry messages, neuron to neuron, within your brain and throughout your body.

When you feel a small stone in your shoe, the neurons in your feet initiate an electrical charge that moves from neuron to neuron until it reaches your brain. There, the message says to your brain, *"Hey, I don't like this stone. Tell my hand to take off my shoe and shake it out."*

Your brain then sends a similar electrical charge—again, along a string of neurons—to your hand, and eventually, the stone ends up back on the ground where it belongs.

These messages travel almost instantaneously through your body, so only a short time elapses between feeling the stone and removing it.

How Neurons Transmit Messages

Electrical charges enter the neuron through one of many appendages that extend out from a neuron. These appendages are called *dendrites*. After passing through the center of the neuron, the message travels through another, much longer appendage called an *axon*.

When the electrical charge reaches the end of the axon, the axon releases a chemical substance called a *neurotransmitter*. This substance transfers the charge across a small gap called a *synapse* to one or more nearby neurons.

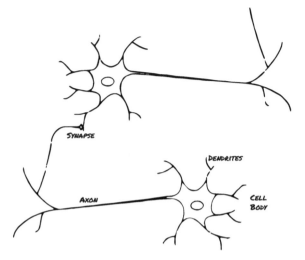

Anatomy of a neuron, including axons, dendrites and synapses

You have billions of neurons, all firing messages at the same time. If enough of these neurons become incapable of transmitting messages, you will begin to experience lost memories, confusion, anger and anxiety.

That stone in your shoe? Imagine knowing something is wrong but having no idea what it is or how to fix it. That's the experience of people with advanced Alzheimer's dementia.

Why Neurons Cease to Function

Alzheimer's dementia has two other hallmarks, discovered from autopsies conducted after a patient's death. Scientists believe that these hallmarks, beta-amyloid plaques and neurofibrillary tangles, instigate the cell death that causes the brain to shrink.

Hallmark #2: Beta-Amyloid Plaques

Under ideal circumstances, beta-amyloid is a protein that scientists think may help protect the brain from infections. A study at Harvard noticed that when microbes threatened healthy cells, beta-amyloid proteins helped to attach carbohydrates to the microbes to incapacitate them.[3]

At these times, beta-amyloid is a friend to the brain.

The beta-amyloid proteins only become a foe when the brain overproduces the proteins or can't eliminate them when their usefulness has ended. At this point, the proteins begin clumping together to form beta-amyloid plaques. The plaques attach to the neuron at the point of the synapse and make it impossible for neurons to transfer messages across that synapse.

How Plaques Form

Here is one likely explanation of why a protein that should help the brain (friend) begins causing so much damage (foe).

Each of the billions of neurons has in its cell membrane a protein called an "Amyloid Precursor Protein" (APP). This protein produces the beta-amyloid in the presence of a fungal or bacterial infection. That means that its first appearance is to protect the brain, not harm it.[4]

Under optimal situations, after the beta-amyloid defeats the infection in the neuronal membrane, the brain gets rid of the beta-amyloid. Job done![5]

But if the brain cannot eliminate the beta-amyloid, it begins to accumulate and clump together. Those clumps are the plaques that are a hallmark of Alzheimer's dementia.

So why can't the brain get rid of the beta-amyloid? To answer that, I'd like to tell you about two garbage collectors.

Every Monday morning, two garbage collectors come to dispose of the used-up beta-amyloid in your brain. These garbage collectors are actually enzymes called α-secretase and y-secretase.

Under normal circumstances, these two enzymes dispose of the fragments created by APP. We don't know exactly what APP does, but at some point it becomes beta-amyloid and emerges from the neuron membrane, sticking out like a little appendage.

This fragment of beta-amyloid needs to be removed from the brain—into the garbage truck and off to the dump.

To do this, our first garbage collector, α-secretase, cuts off a piece of the beta-amyloid, and then the y-secretase follows suit—snip, snip in quick sequence. The two fragments then escape into the fluid around the neuron and are carried away, never to be seen again.

Our two garbage collectors work well together. They have the necessary training and experience and are overall good people.[6]

Some days, however, α-secretase fails to show up and β-secretase comes instead. β-secretase is neither experienced nor competent, and it cuts off a big fragment of APP that is much too big to be carried away and out of the brain.

The fragments are very sticky, and they begin to clump together on the outside of the neuron's wall. These become the dreaded beta-amyloid plaques.[7]

The poor neuron! How can it do its work with these bulbous growths gumming up its synapse?

When neuron can no longer do its work, the brain somehow signals the neuron that it has outlived its usefulness. In response, tau tangles—the last hallmark of Alzheimer's dementia—form in the cell. These tau tangles become a death sentence for the cell.

Hallmark #3: Tau Tangles

Inside of each neuron, we have a remarkable network of fibers that act as a simple skeleton for the neurons and as a transport system inside the neuron. These fibers carry messages inside the neuron from one end to the other end, where the signals will cross the synapse to another neuron.

It might help to think of these fibers as flexible pipes. Around these pipes is a protective cord made up of tau proteins, holding the network together.

After beta-amyloid plaques accumulate outside of the neurons, for some reason, the tau protein unravels from around the network of fibers and the tubes no longer hold together.

The unraveled tau protein gets knotted up, forming a neurofibrillary tangle, or tau tangle. These tangles choke off the neuron from inside, making it impossible for the neuron to survive.[8]

Neuroinflammation Follows Plaques and Tangles

The brain perceives the plaques and tangles as dangerous threats, so inflammation in the brain (*neuroinflammation*) follows cell death like a bad smell.

A cascade of other processes follows, some of which can lead to additional plaque and tangle formation, further cell damage, and many more problems related to dementia.

How Alzheimer's Dementia Advances Through the Brain

Alzheimer's dementia has a fairly predictable journey of damage through the brain:

1. **Memory:** The damage that beta-amyloid plaques

and tau tangles do to neurons seems to occur first in the hippocampus, the center of memory in the brain.

2. **Cell damage:** The plaques and tangles spread from the hippocampus to other parts of the brain, which results in further cell (neuron) damage and death.

3. **Executive function:** When the plaques and tangles reach the frontal cortex—the executive function of the brain—the brain loses its ability to reason, understand concepts or make decisions.

4. **Language:** Soon language declines, and patients have difficulty finding the right words. This is when people begin to suspect Alzheimer's dementia.

5. **Final Decline:** Eventually, the damage from plaques and tangles is so extensive that the patient enters a vegetative state and finally dies.

Optimal Brain Health

For years, researchers have been seeking a way to eliminate beta-amyloid plaques. They hope this will reverse the process of Alzheimer's dementia. I hope one day these researchers succeed.

This is the old model for treating Alzheimer's dementia because it focuses on what happens in the brain. I will discuss it in the next chapter.

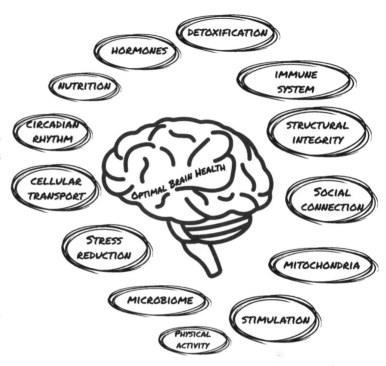

Help your body, help your brain!

I am offering you a new approach. I cannot guarantee a cure from Alzheimer's, but I can offer many ways to reduce your risk of dementia, especially Alzheimer's dementia. If you act on these suggestions, you have a good chance of achieving optimal brain health.

Chapter 2

Old and New Models of Alzheimer's Treatment

> *"Though the problems of the world are increasingly complex, the solutions remain embarrassingly simple."*
>
> *- Bill Mollison*

The Older Model for Treating Alzheimer's

If someone has chest pain that persists, that person will see a heart doctor. The doctor does tests, diagnoses the problem and presents a plan of care that might include medication, therapy, lifestyle changes or surgery.

Vision problems? An eye doctor does tests, diagnoses and prescribes treatment—often a pair of glasses or contacts.

Fever with a sore throat? The doctor does an examination, makes a diagnosis and then prescribes treatment, usually antibiotics.

Symptoms. Diagnosis. Prescription. And then a return to health.

This is the model of medical treatment that most of us expect and even desire, but it doesn't work well with a chronic disease like Alzheimer's dementia.

Let's work through the process.

Symptoms

We now know that neuron damage and death begins long before symptoms appear, so addressing Alzheimer's dementia after symptoms occur is too late.

Also, many people with symptoms of Alzheimer's delay going to a doctor and may try to avoid it altogether.

After all, the symptoms may disappear, right? Besides, I don't want to risk my driver's license, my dog, my independence, and what will people think when they hear I have Alzheimer's?

For these and other reasons, people with memory loss usually see a doctor only after a family member notices a decline and insists they get their forgetfulness checked out.

Diagnosis

Diagnosis is extremely difficult with Alzheimer's dementia. The doctor will look for other dementia-related diseases which can be diagnosed, but if none emerges, the doctor has to suspect Alzheimer's. He or she will gather anecdotal evidence from family members and give the patient memory and other cognitive tests.

But any diagnosis of Alzheimer's dementia is essentially speculative, with certainty growing in the coming years.

Treatment

With Alzheimer's dementia, there is no medication plan that can effectively reduce or eliminate symptoms once those symptoms appear.

Return to health

This isn't possible. Once Alzheimer's has been diagnosed under this old model of treatment, further deterioration is inevitable, leading eventually to decline, dependency and death.

The New Preventive Model for Alzheimer's

Our bodies are very complex. The cells, tissues and organs throughout our bodies all work together in harmony. In medicine, we tend to divide all these systems for the sake of our education. However, dementia is a complex, whole-body problem and is not only a brain problem.

I am convinced that many of the root causes of dementia begin far beyond the confines of our brains, and we will be able to prevent dementia only when we treat the body as an integrated whole.

This idea that dementia originates outside the brain is a new approach to Alzheimer's dementia, a new lens through which we view dementia.

What lifestyle choices might contribute to dementia? Scientists are considering inflammatory

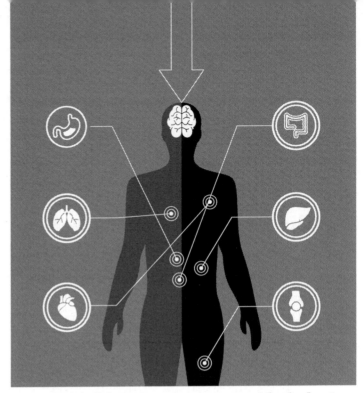

A new model: Dementia starts outside the brain

food, poor sleep, stress, inactivity, toxins and an unhealthy gut. These problems outside the brain may be causing the memory loss and cell death that are hallmarks of Alzheimer's dementia. If so, this is good news because it offers hope that you can control your future.

In this book, I have gathered information on problems *outside* the brain that may contribute to neuron damage. I hope you can use this information to shore up your defenses against Alzheimer's and that, as you modify your lifestyle choices, your brain—and your life—will thrive.

Preliminary Steps That Will Help You Reduce Your Risk of Alzheimer's

1. Widen your understanding of Alzheimer's.

Instead of something that happens in the brain, I suggest you think of Alzheimer's as a metabolic process that occurs in your body, and that this process has a neurological presentation. The metabolic process occurs because of lifestyle choices.

The problem becomes even more urgent when we realize the metabolic process affects more than just the brain. It alters the entire network of cells in our organs.

Accepting this new perspective will empower us to create and enact strategies that will reduce our risk of Alzheimer's.

2. You need your own, personalized plan.

Each of us is unique. We have different fingerprints, different DNA, different life experiences and different personalities. So although our many different preventive treatment plans will have overlapping elements (the modifiable lifestyle choices that I discuss in **Sections 2 and 3** of this book), your personal plan for reducing your risks will be different than mine.

If you are going to make this work, you will need to consider all the lifestyle choices discussed in this book. These choices include nutrition, exercise, detoxifying, learning, and more. You will need to evaluate your current lifestyle and habits to isolate areas of potential problems, then create your own plan for reducing your

We each need a personal Dementia Action Plan

risk of Alzheimer's, adding variables as you see fit.

3. Now is the time to think about Alzheimer's.

We now know that cognitive decline begins decades before we first notice it. We also understand factors that influence our likelihood of experiencing Alzheimer's.

The harm in our brains that leads to dementia occurs over a long period. If we don't act promptly, that damage will negatively impact our lives—and may even end them.

COGNITIVE AND PHYSICAL ABILITIES ▲

PRE-DEMENTIA PHASE
20 years before first symptoms

*Measurable damage occurring in the brain,
but no apparent symptoms at this stage other than
occasional senior moments.*

**This is the golden time to reduce your risk
of Alzheimer's dementia.**

MILD COGNITIVE IMPAIRMENT

Symptoms appear but do not significantly interfere with everyday activities

Still time to reduce your risk

ALZHEIMER'S DEMENTIA

Increasing confusion, memory loss, inability to reason and plan, dependence, leading to death

Pre-death decline

DEMENTIA PROGRESSION ▶

Progression of damage in the brain from pre-dementia to Alzheimer's and death.

Remember, one in three seniors dies with Alzheimer's or another form of dementia.[9] Now is the time to act!

4. *You have the power to create overall health and regeneration.*

What follows is an extremely simplified picture of why we die. It illustrates the extent to which lifestyle choices affect our ability to think.

Your body has trillions of cells. Imagine that at any given second, each cell is trying to survive by balancing two opposite forces—regeneration and degeneration.

The forces of degeneration include accidents, trauma, illness, stress, sleep deprivation and toxins. The forces of regeneration include all the good things we provide to help our cells stay healthy—clean air, healthy food and exercise.

Our choices and experiences affect whether degeneration or regeneration is winning in the cells in our body and our brain.

If the regenerative forces are winning in our brain, then our thinking is sharp and vibrant, and we can look forward to success and learning and wisdom.

But if the degenerative forces start winning, then our ability to think declines and we feel anxious, tired, weak and sad, and eventually the symptoms of Alzheimer's appear.

As the cell deaths accumulate, our ability to sustain life diminishes, and eventually we die.

The choices you make every hour, every day, help to support regeneration. I can't guarantee that the plan you create to reduce your risk of Alzheimer's will prevent, reverse or cure Alzheimer's. But if you use these building blocks, you will be healthier as you eliminate dementia-related risk factors.

Some Final Words on Your Dementia Action Plan

The options in this book will probably seem overwhelming. Please—please—set your own pace for making changes. You are starting a journey with many steps, but you get to choose those steps and the speed at which you take them.

No matter what your plan turns out to be, through it all you'll need determination and discipline, but—*this is the good news*—the rewards will be great because you'll not only increase your chance of avoiding Alzheimer's, you'll also improve your overall health.

Start now and keep moving toward your personalized goals. You **do** have the power to tip the balance of your life toward the side of health.

I wish you well!

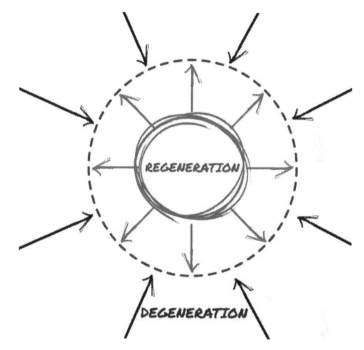

Regenerative and degenerative forces are at work in your body all the time.

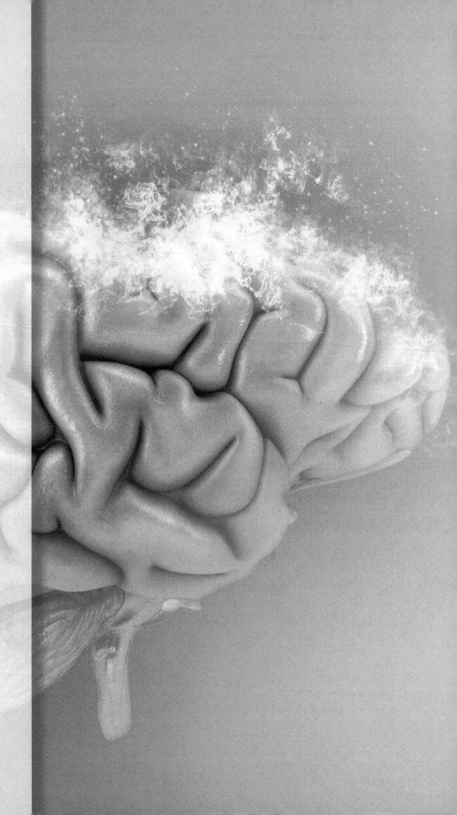

Chapter 3
Inflammation and Dementia

**Dementia,
Brain on Fire**

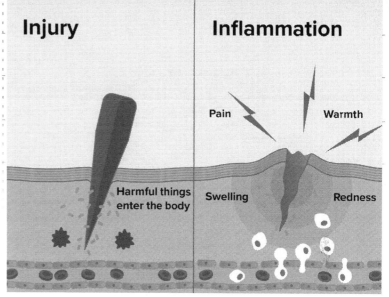

Injury · **Inflammation**

Pain · Warmth

Harmful things enter the body · Swelling · Redness

An inflammatory response to injury

Acute Inflammation—Friend

Acute inflammation is a short-term immune response. When you get a bee sting or bump on your head, your body rushes plasma and white blood cells to the injured tissue. A warm, red bump appears. That bump is the inflammation.

Think of fire trucks and ambulances showing up in response to a 911 call, or maybe even police cars and a SWAT team. The inflammation you see is like that response. Inflammation rushes to the scene to eliminate a threat to your health.[10]

With *acute inflammation,* the immune response does its work and then, like the responders, leaves the scene. The site of inflammation calms down, and the body returns to normal.

This inflammation is a friend because it both starts and *ends.*

Chronic Inflammation—Foe

There's another kind of inflammation called *chronic inflammation* that occurs when the threat lingers, gets repeated or never goes away.

When that happens, the immune response goes a little crazy and starts killing healthy cells in its desperate attempt to remove the primary threat.

Because the inflammation never goes away, it becomes a foe. From the original site of the threat, the inflammation spreads throughout the body, resulting in widespread damage.

Chronic inflammation contributes to many chronic diseases like diabetes, arthritis, kidney diseases, fibromyalgia, Crohn's disease and heart diseases.[11]

In fact, I believe that *every* chronic disease has some component of inflammation—including Alzheimer's.

I previously described acute inflammation as a SWAT response. Chronic inflammation is more akin to a destructive, seemingly endless war. During a war, nothing about life is normal, and in extreme cases, essential services like water, electricity, education and food transport stop. And yet somehow, life must go on.

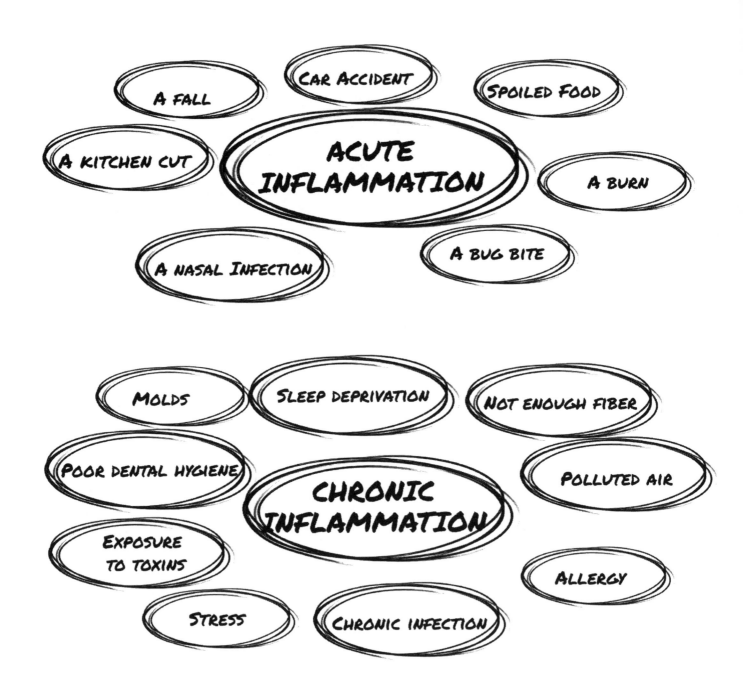

In the same way, someone with a chronic disease must carry on as well, in spite of the pain, problems, lack of energy and discomfort.

The Brain's Primary Immune System

What about the brain? Does inflammation occur in the brain? Does chronic inflammation?

To answer this, first I need to explain a little more about the brain's unique immune system.

Years ago, when scientists injected blue dye into the bloodstream of an animal, they discovered that tissues throughout the body turned blue except in the brain and spinal cord. The dye could not get out of the blood vessels into the brain's tissue.

They concluded that blood vessels in the brain and spinal cord must have a special protective layer surrounding them. This protective layer kept the blue dye from exiting the blood vessels and entering the brain's tissues.

They called this protective layer the **blood-brain barrier**. The cells in this layer are packed closely together. When functioning properly, they keep dangerous pathogens like bacteria and viruses out of your brain, as well as toxins and other damaging substances.

It occurred to the scientists that the blood-brain barrier also kept out the immune cells that circulate throughout the rest of the body's blood vessels. Did that mean the brain didn't need an immune system?

Absolutely not! The brain actually has its own, very effective immune system. This system has specialized immune cells called **microglia** which appear nowhere else in the body. At the first sign of danger, microglia attack just as immune cells do elsewhere in the body.

A Secondary Way to Protect the Brain

For a while scientists assumed that with its own immune system, the brain made no use of the body's regular immune system.

But does it make sense that the most critical organ in your body, the command post and center for all thought, decision, action and memory would limit itself when it comes to immune responses? Based on evidence from recent research, scientists are answering that question with a resounding, *"No!"*

Scientists now acknowledge that in cases of infection or injury, the brain does accumulate immune cells from the peripheral immune system. Some scientists also believe that the brain uses peripheral immune cells even under normal circumstances.[12]

But if the blood vessels' blood-brain barrier keeps immune cells from entering the brain's tissues, how do these cells enter the brain?

They appear to enter through the three membranes that surround the brain: the pia mater, the arachnoid membrane and the outer dura mater. They show up especially when a healthy individual's brain becomes compromised in some way, such as during extreme stress, infection in the brain or the presence of toxins.[13]

Just as elsewhere in the body, acute inflammation (friend) is part of the brain's immune response to a threat. When a threat lingers or overwhelms the brain, chronic neuroinflammation occurs (foe).[14]

Threats to the Brain

These threats include a traumatic brain injury from a car accident, assault or fall. The inflammation may also result from stress caused by troubles in your life.

In other cases, the blood-brain barrier becomes compromised. The problem might come from a leaky gut, air pollution, the wrong fats, cardiovascular weakness, too much sugar or any of the other problems presented in this book. Once compromised, the blood-brain barrier starts allowing toxins, bacteria, viruses and other threats to enter the brain.[15]

Understandably, the brain goes on alert, calling out both its own immune system (microglia) and the immune system from the rest of the body.

In the face of a lingering or recurring threat, uncontrolled inflammation damages healthy neurons.[16] As you know by now, cell damage and death harm your ability to think, reason and remember.

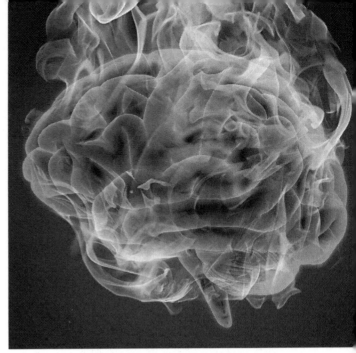

Chronic neuroinflammation:
A contributing factor to Alzheimer's?

Alzheimer's and Neuroinflammation

We don't have to guess about the relationship of neuroinflammation and Alzheimer's dementia. In autopsies, we see an abundance of activated microglia cells in the brains of people who had Alzheimer's.[17] So neuroinflammation has become another hallmark of Alzheimer's.

But is neuroinflammation the *result* of Alzheimer's or the *cause* of Alzheimer's?

In the past, scientists assumed that Alzheimer's occurred first and inflammation followed. Today, more and more scientists believe that inflammation is driving the disease—the inflammation occurs first, and then cognitive damage follows.

Probably, both are true to some extent. The inflammatory processes in the brain are incredibly complex, and we are just beginning to understand them.

Let's just say this: If you want to keep your brain healthy, you need to limit whatever contributes to inflammation in your brain.

So How Can I Reduce Neuroinflammation?

Simple answer: Get the garbage out of your life.

This garbage includes smoking, poor sleep habits, stress, unhealthy foods and drinks, a sedentary lifestyle, extra body weight and the other modifiable lifestyle changes I discuss in the next section of the book.

Then replace each of these with better alternatives. This book explains how.

To succeed, you will need many small steps in the right direction. You will have missteps, encounter obstacles, rough roads, and get distracted, but as long as you continue heading in the right direction, you will improve your health and reduce your risk of Alzheimer's. Take your time and keep moving forward.

Remember, your body wants to thrive. It wants to be healthy, vibrant, and full of energy. If you work with your body, your body will reward you.

There's no set deadlines, no prescribed set of steps. Instead, you will need to design your own plan for better health—what to work on first, second and third—and to what extent.

Perhaps you already have excellent, healthy nutrition, but quality sleep is a problem. Maybe you exercise religiously but can't seem to give up sugar. Perhaps you have never smoked, but you're addicted to soft drinks. Decide for yourself what lifestyle changes to work on and in what order.

In my own life I have found that if I make a change for just 90 days, I feel so much better that I keep going. And because so much of your health is connected, when you make that one change, you'll discover that other aspects of your health have improved as well.

It works great!

Before explaining the modifiable lifestyle changes you can make, I want to inform you of one more very exciting concept called *epigenetics*. I hope you will consider epigenetics as an ally in your fight against Alzheimer's.

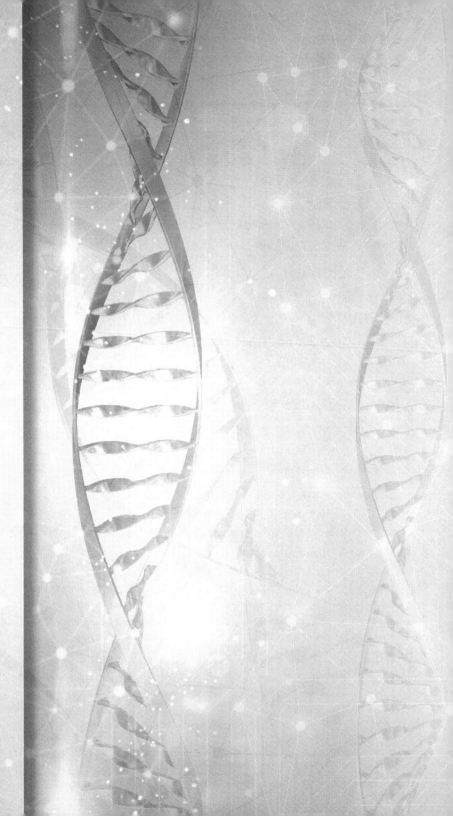

Chapter 4

Genes and Dementia

*Your genes are
not your destiny.*

A Clarification

In this chapter, I am not discussing genetics related to Familial Alzheimer's Disease (FAD). FAD is entirely passed down through the family, and its cause is genetic. It is exceedingly rare and accounts for only 2-3% of all cases of Alzheimer's.[18]

Instead, I will discuss genetic connections related to more typical kinds of Alzheimer's dementia.

Your Genes and Alzheimer's

Your DNA stores all the instructions your cells need to do their work, grow, develop, function and reproduce. You get this DNA at conception, and except in the most adverse circumstances (such as exposure to dangerously high levels of radiation), the code doesn't change.

Does this mean your future is set if you have a parent who died from Alzheimer's dementia? Do you have somewhere in your genetic code an indelible mark that says, *"This person will get Alzheimer's?"*

Right up front, I say: ***No! This is not true.***

Except for the rare instances of Familial Alzheimer's Disease discussed earlier, your genes are not your destiny.

That's because even though DNA code cannot change, the *expression* of your genes can definitely change based on your lifestyle choices.

Whatever you eat, drink, touch, breathe or think dynamically affects your metabolic pathways, and your metabolic pathways affect the expression of your genes.

Some people compare this process to playing the piano. Your DNA has certain keys on the keyboard, in a certain order.

Your lifestyle choices determine what keys get played. Some of those choices contribute to Alzheimer's—such as poor sleep and smoking. Others work against Alzheimer's—such as plant-based diet and exercise. So your lifestyle choices can reduce your risk of Alzheimer's.

We call the ability of genes to change their expression *epigenetics*. Epigenetics offers you a measure of control over whether you get Alzheimer's.

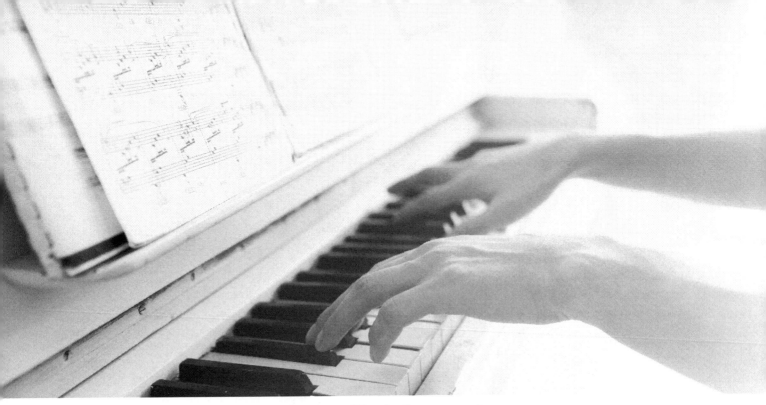

Genes are like the keys on a piano.
Your lifestyle choices determine what keys get played.

If you have a parent who died from Alzheimer's you have a statistically higher risk of Alzheimer's. This does not mean you are guaranteed to get the disease.

In this case, however, making and adhering to a Dementia Action Plan is all the more important for you. The modifiable lifestyle changes you address in your Action Plan can potentially override that greater risk.

Evidence from a Tribe in Nigeria

One of the many genes associated with Alzheimer's is the ApoE4 gene. Nigerian people have the highest observed frequency of the ApoE4 gene. They also have the lowest rate of Alzheimer's on the globe.

We believe their choices—in other words, the way they are "playing" the keys in their genetic code—silence the ApoE4 gene while amplifying other protective genes. [19]

The typical Nigerian lifestyle includes a diet based on fruits and vegetables, great exercise and sleep and many other healthy choices, with very little of the "garbage" that can contribute to Alzheimer's.

Evidence from Twin Studies

Twins share 100% of their genes, so it might seem like the expression of those genes would also be identical. In fact, twins often share many surprising similarities.

One set of twins, separated at birth but reunited at age 39, discovered they both had terrible migraines, chewed their fingernails, drove light blue Chevrolets and smoked Salem cigarettes.

Both also previously worked at McDonald's and as part-time deputy sheriffs. They had been poor in spelling and math. One of the twins named his first son James Alan, and the other named his first son James Allan. Both named their pet dogs "Toy."

The two men both married women named Linda, but later divorced, and then both remarried women named Betty.[20]

If genes are like a piano and DNA a keyboard, these two men played pretty much the same song!

And yet I still maintain that genes are not your destiny because not all identical twins grow into cookie cutter versions of each other.

Only 50% of twins share schizophrenia, for example, which has a definite genetic component. Identical twins can be different heights—the average difference is 2 inches. One may develop breast cancer and the other not, one may have severe autism and the other only mild and only one may develop diabetes.

With these identical twins, scientists believe that environmental factors made the difference. Perhaps only one twin smoked. Perhaps they had different diets and physical activity levels. One may have experienced a traumatic injury or a particularly severe case of chicken pox.

Differences can also occur prenatally, such as one twin having a larger placenta than the other. Sometimes a radical difference can happen very early in life because of surgery following a trauma.

All these differences occur because the genes have been expressed differently. As twins age, the possible differences multiply.

But what about Alzheimer's?

One twin study examined Alzheimer's specifically. Peter Miller in *National Geographic* tells about a pair of identical twins. One developed early-onset Alzheimer's and one still showed no symptoms of the illness eight years later.[21]

Epigenetics offers the only reasonable explanation for this. Something, sometime—and possibly over a long period—changed the genetic expression of the twin without Alzheimer's so that she has been able to avoid getting the disease.

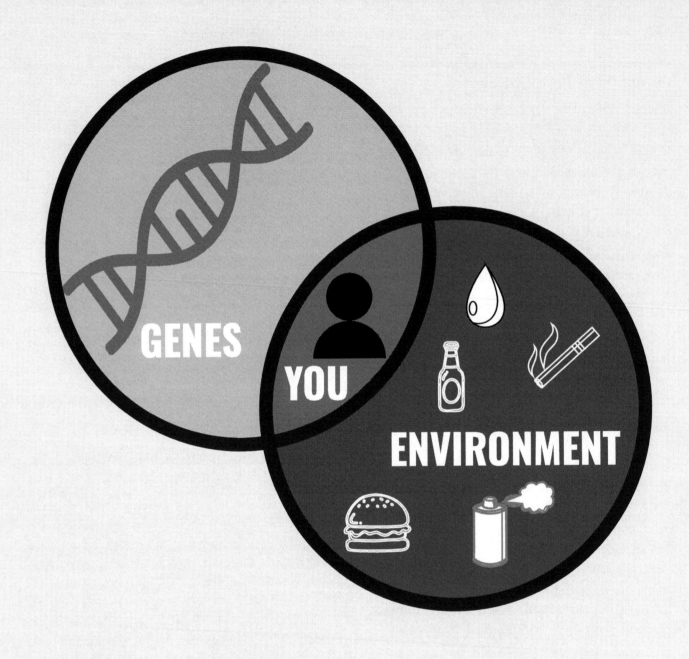

Your genetic code and your lifestyle choices determine the expression of your genes.

Your risk of Alzheimer's is not a game of slots. You control the odds through your choices.

A Source of Hope

As our understanding of epigenetics develops, perhaps one day we will be able to hack epigenetics and gene expression to avoid Alzheimer's as this identical twin did. This will not be easy because chronic diseases like Alzheimer's are almost certainly controlled by more than one gene and possibly several series of genes.

A chronic disease is like a box, but instead of a simple key to open the box—or a simple pill to take—you need to figure out a complex code that involves your environment, your genome, your microbiome (gut) and many other variables.

The boxes are different for heart disease, diabetes, Parkinson's, Alzheimer's, multiple sclerosis and other chronic diseases.

Many thanks to the researchers and scientists who are trying to unlock the codes for these diseases. As Peter Miller says, "someday epigenetic mistakes will be as simple to repair as a piano that's out of tune."[22]

In the meantime, you can tilt the odds in your favor by making modifiable lifestyle changes that will reduce your risk of getting Alzheimer's and improve your overall health.

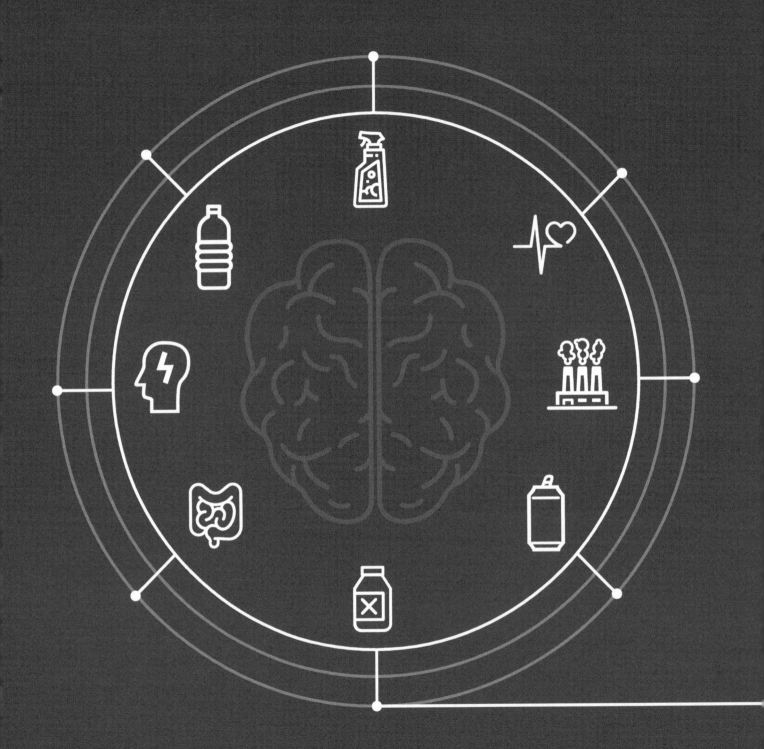

Section 2

Rid Your Life of Dementia-Related Risks

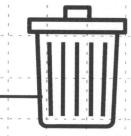

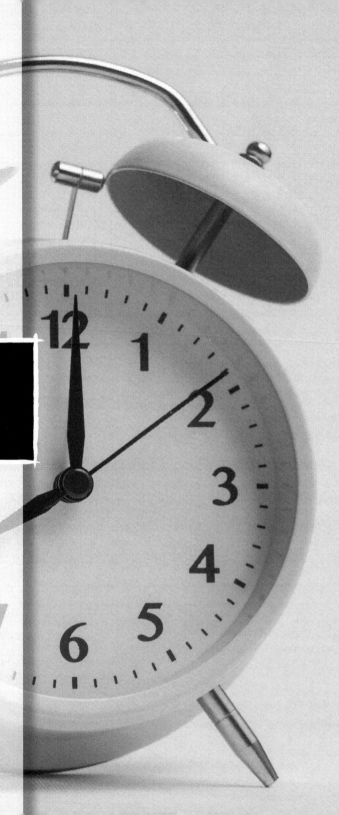

Chapter 5

Rid Your Body of Sleep Deprivation

Sleep—the most powerful anti-aging medicine

When it comes to your Dementia Action Plan, I consider ensuring high-quality sleep the first and foremost modifiable lifestyle change you need to make. It's easy to deprive yourself of sleep, and even easier for it to become a habit, but the harm this does to your body, mind and emotions is extreme.

Nature follows a rhythm—summer follows spring, night follows day.

Your body has a rhythm as well, a cycle that occurs roughly every 24 hours. We call this your circadian rhythm (in Latin *circa* means around and *dies* means day). This rhythm controls your sleep, wakefulness and digestion.

Chemicals in your body—neurotransmitters, hormones and other chemicals—control this rhythm. When you wake up, your norepinephrine, dopamine, serotonin and acetylcholine all go up, and when you want to sleep, your GABA and melatonin take over.[23]

The Effects of Sleep Deprivation

For all this to work well, you need regular and ample sleep. Each of us is different, so the amount of sleep we need varies. Some of us need as little as seven hours,

some as much as nine hours. But if you get either too much or too little sleep, you'll feel foggy the next day. I feel most rested after 7-1/2 hours of sleep every night.

Unfortunately, more than a third of people in United States are not getting enough sleep. If you are one of them, this could result from your evening routines, insomnia, diseases, pain, anxiety, depression or a sleep disorder called sleep apnea (more on this later).

Your brain recognizes that this lack of sleep is a severe threat to your health, and it responds as it always does to a threat, with an inflammatory immune response.

If sustained, the resulting inflammation contributes to a host of health problems, including diabetes, heart trouble, mental problems and damaging expressions of genes throughout your body.

I ignored this part of my health for ten years while I worked the night shift in the emergency room, and I paid a heavy price for it. The disturbances to my circadian rhythm caused significant mental, physical and social problems in my life.

You don't have to work a night shift to know how

much sleep deprivation can affect your life. One late night, and you'll be forgetful the next day. Keep it up and you'll have trouble controlling your emotions and behavior.

I'm sure you've experienced this.

Sleep Deprivation and the Brain

The effects of sleep deprivation on the brain are profound and far-reaching.

First, the inflammation that results from a lack of sleep causes a destructive chain reaction in the brain. This reaction begins when the inflammation makes the blood-brain barrier more porous. This allows more toxins and other dangerous substances to pass from your bloodstream into your brain.[24]

The presence of these invaders triggers even more inflammation in the brain. This leads to more damage to the blood-brain barrier, and more damage to your brain. Your weary brain can't keep up, and your lack of sleep makes it even worse, as you'll see.

Even if nothing else was happening in the brain as you sleep, this damage alone would make sleep extremely important to your cognitive health.

But something else *is* happening in the brain as you sleep. In fact, sleep is probably the most important time of the day for your cognitive health.

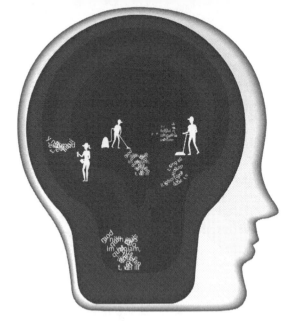

Your brain has a dedicated janitorial service that works while you sleep.

What the Brain Does During Sleep

Your Brain's Waste Management System

When your immune cells try to reconcile the inflammation that occurs in your brain, the immune cells damage more than just the blood-brain barrier. They also cause collateral damage to nearby cells, leading to cell destruction and death. If the brain doesn't remove those damaged cells, they will eventually lead to even more inflammation.

Fortunately, your brain has a five-star waste management system. This *glymphatic system* involves billions of cells called glial cells that infiltrate every part of the brain, surrounding all the neurons and synapses.[25]

When working correctly, the glymphatic system uses the fluid in the brain (the cerebrospinal fluid, or CSF) to sweep away the trash left over from inflammatory responses. It also removes toxins, bacteria and other unwanted substances.

A strong glymphatic system, therefore, is essential to your overall brain health and crucial to ridding the brain of the damage that results in inflammation.

One problem: You need ample deep sleep for this crew to work well. In fact, 60% of their work happens during deep sleep.[26]

Scientists think this is because your brain has so much else to do during the day. Also, during waking hours, noradrenaline inhibits the glymphatic system. Noradrenaline's activity during sleep is much lower, allowing for excellent waste management.

When you don't get enough sleep, however, the noradrenaline stays high, and your glymphatic system can't do its job. Think of an office building where no one ever goes home so that the janitorial crew can't get its work done. Your brain needs you to sleep!

One more analogy: Imagine a hiker who has gravel in her shoes. She's in pain. The gravel slows her down. It distracts her, and she becomes curt and unfriendly to her companions. That's not all. The gravel is shredding the skin on her feet, and she suffers long-term damage.

If you don't get enough sleep, you'll be like that hiker. You'll not only experience foggy thinking and emotional difficulties. You'll also do long-term damage to your brain.

If you want to avoid Alzheimer's, you need sleep.

Other Benefits of Sleep

During deep sleep, your brain readjusts itself, making sense of your social and psychological experiences from the day. How often have you awakened at 4:00 or 5:00 in the morning and remembered something you needed to do? Without adequate sleep, your brain will miss out on this chance to organize itself.

Sleep also regulates your appetite—which is why poor sleep and weight gain are often linked.

Other benefits of good sleep include:

- Decreased risk of stroke
- Better sex
- Less infection
- Less stress

With so many benefits, it's easy to see why better sleep is so important to your well-being. It will also profoundly reduce your risk of Alzheimer's dementia. The time to banish sleep deprivation from your life is now!

How to improve your sleep

 - *Avoid heavy, pro-inflammatory meals and snacks, especially in the evening:* These include foods high in sugar, baked and fried foods, and most processed foods. (See Chapters 10 and 11.)

• ***Get some morning sunshine:*** This lets your body know it's time to be awake. It's best to get this sunshine between 6:30 and 8:30 in the morning. You could accomplish this with a 30-minute morning walk, or you could sit outside while drinking a cup of coffee. If your routine makes all this impossible, you could also purchase a light that simulates sunshine to sit on your desk or light therapy glasses you can wear.

 • ***Get some exercise:*** A 30-minute walk will help. But limit any vigorous exercise to three or four hours before trying to sleep.

 • ***Keep yourself hydrated:*** Especially during the daytime because night-time drinking could cause you to wake up during the night to relieve yourself.

 • ***Don't take naps:*** Especially in the afternoon or early evening. You can overcome an afternoon "slump" by avoiding carbohydrates at lunch, taking a short walk, drinking a glass of water or splashing water on your face.

 • ***Avoid caffeine*** in the afternoon, including chocolate and pain relievers that include caffeine. If you still have trouble, limit all caffeine to the hours before 9:00 a.m.

 • ***Turn off screens 30-60 minutes before bedtime:*** You should also dim your other lights. The blue light from TVs, computers, tablets, fluorescent bulbs and cell phones inhibits your body's production of melatonin, affecting your natural sleep rhythms.

To block blue light:

 • ***Wear amber-colored glasses*** during the crucial 30-60 minutes before going to bed. Studies have shown that the amber lenses help produce melatonin as much as if the room were completely dark. Look for glasses that cut out almost all the blue light.

 • ***Install amber-colored light bulbs*** in your living room and bedroom.

• ***Turn on blue-light filters*** on your computer, tablet and cell phone an hour before sleep. You can find many apps for blue-light filters.

 • ***Have only a light snack after dinner, at least an hour before bed:*** Consume heavier foods earlier in the day.

 • ***Avoid alcohol:*** After the initial effects of your "nightcap" wear off, alcohol will make you wake up more often during the night.

 • ***Avoid nicotine:*** It's a stimulant and can inhibit sleep.

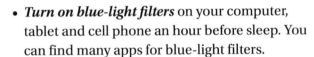 • ***Make your bedroom as comfortable as possible:*** It should be quiet, dark, cool and free of distractions. A fan, air-conditioner or white

noise machine can eliminate annoying sounds.

- **If your mind is rushing:** Make a few notes on whatever you're thinking about, and then take a warm (not hot) bath, preferably with lights lowered.

- **Meditate, pray or listen to calming music:** These can calm the mind and stop it from racing. These also help you become more intentional with your breathing, which encourages sleep. You might also take part in a mindful form of movement that relieves stress and calms your mind.

Try some age-old remedies:

- **Chamomile tea** decreases anxiety and insomnia. 200-1000 mg daily has been shown to reduce anxiety in clinical research.

- **Passionflower** has been used for centuries by Native Americans. Passionflower leaves can be used to make tea which reduces insomnia, anxiety and pain.

- **Valerian extracts** taken a few hours before bedtime may improve your sleep.

- **Melatonin**, available over the counter, will improve your sleep patterns and quality. I recommend starting with 1 mg each evening and increasing this to at maximum of 3 mg. (Review this with your doctor.)

- **Aromatherapy with lavender or rosemary** will decrease your cortisol and stress and will enhance your healthy sleep patterns. You can rub lavender oil under your nose as aromatherapy or spray your pillow with lavender.

- **A warm bath**: My wife combines 2 cups of Epsom salts, 1 ½ cups of baking soda and 15 drops of lavender oil, pours it into a warm bath and soaks for 20-30 minutes.

- **Sex and orgasm** reboot your brain computer, reducing stress and improving your sleep.

Seek help if your sleeplessness lasts more than a month. There might be a medical cause. Your doctor may be able to help.

One More Issue: Sleep Apnea

Sleep apnea is a disorder that interrupts a person's breathing during sleep. Something may be blocking the airway, or the brain may not be signaling the muscles to breathe. The incidence of sleep apnea is rising at an alarming rate, often occurring in parallel to other chronic illnesses. Here are two ways sleep apnea damages your brain:

1. **Sleep apnea keeps you from sleeping well because when you stop breathing, your body reacts by startling you awake.** Some people with sleep

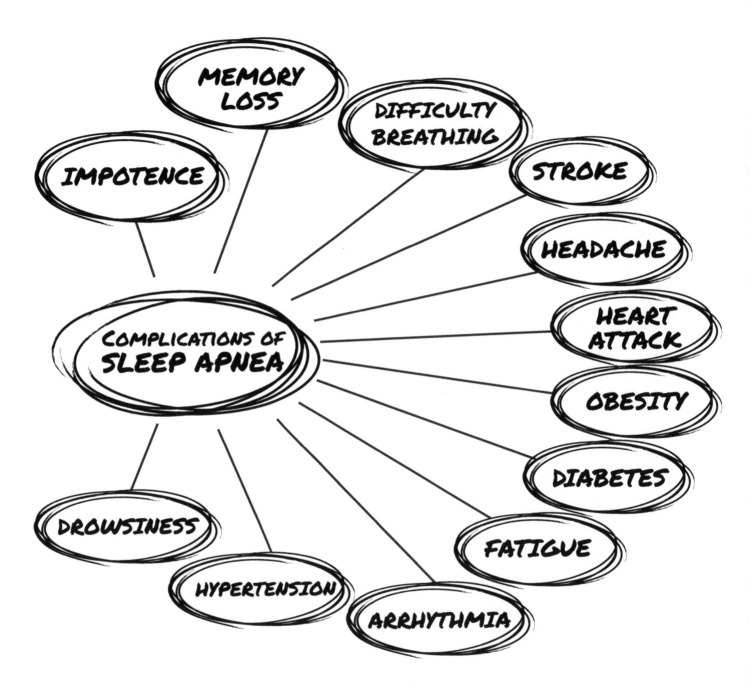

Sleep apnea contributes to many problems.

apnea have 75-100 episodes like this every night, seriously disturbing their sleep. This impedes your brain's ability to clean out debris, toxins and other unwanted substances.

2. ***It deprives your brain of oxygen, which is necessary for life and health.*** The few moments you are not sleeping can have a severe effect on your brain cells, especially the mitochondria inside the cells that provide energy. If these energy factories in the cells do not have sufficient oxygen, your brain, eyes and muscles suffer the most.

Sleep apnea creates a cascade of problems that contribute to Alzheimer's. If you have trouble sleeping, and especially if you are prone to snoring, get checked for sleep apnea.

During the months and years of my worst health, I suffered from sleep apnea. I was constantly tired.

I had sore muscles and frequently experienced eye infections. Finally, I was prescribed a continuous positive airway pressure (CPAP) machine to help me breathe better in sleep. It took a while to get used to the machine, but it was worth it because I needed it to function normally during the day.

Many people have trouble adjusting to a CPAP machine, but those who do never want to sleep without it. It changes their lives.[27]

Better Sleep Today... Better Day Tomorrow!

Poor sleep is a chronic, 24-hour lifestyle problem resulting from choices during the day and night. Decide what changes to make first, then start slow and go forward.

You will be glad you did.

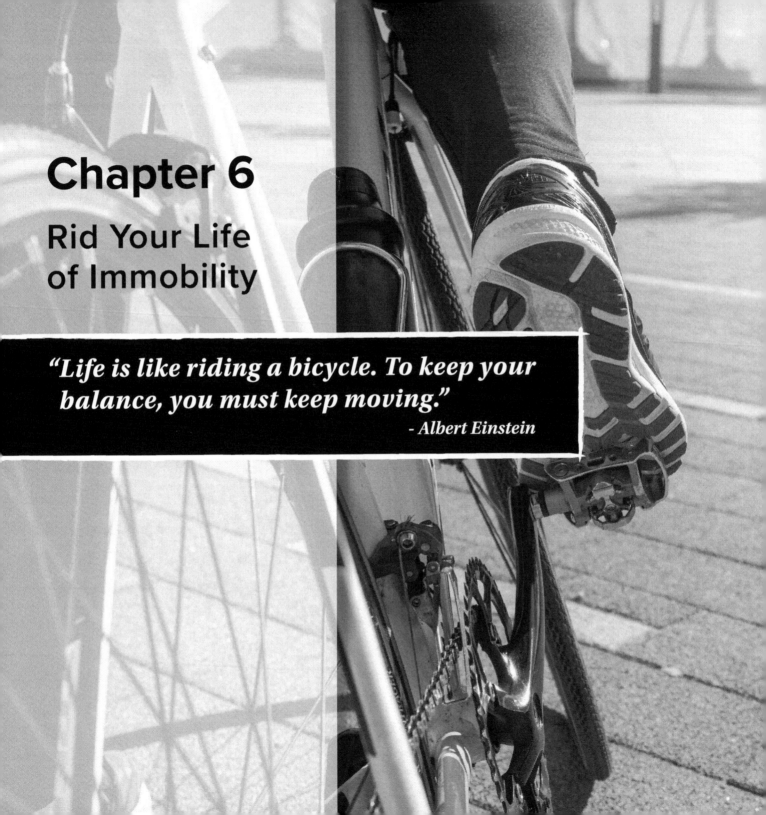

Chapter 6

Rid Your Life of Immobility

"Life is like riding a bicycle. To keep your balance, you must keep moving."

— Albert Einstein

When I was so sick, I always took the elevator—even for one floor. I sat at my computer for hours and drove around the corner to pick up something from the store. Doing so little, why was I so tired?

After deciding to improve my health, increasing my movement was one of the first changes I made. I began by taking a short walk which wore me out horribly, but my body soon adjusted and I began to crave movement. Now movement is a normal part of my life, and I hope it will be for you as well.

You'll be amazed how much better you feel.

But please, this is very important: Before making any changes to your exercise routines, check with your doctor.

Healthy Heart

Perhaps the most significant benefit of exercise you'll see is better circulation. Exercise strengthens your heart, enabling it to pump more blood to your body.

In the brain, blood is the source of nutrients and oxygen, so getting too little blood eventually adds up to big problems. Exercise delivers a healthy feast to your brain, making it very happy. *Happy heart, happy brain.*

Exercise and Inflammation

Exercise done correctly can decrease chronic inflammation because it strengthens your body's immune response, helping it to defeat whatever causes chronic inflammation in the first place.

Just 20-30 minutes of moderate exercise, such as brisk walking, will trigger this anti-inflammatory cellular response.[28] If you move this much, you are likely to live longer, and if you don't, you are likely to die younger. So let's get moving!

But wait! Doesn't exercise cause inflammation? Isn't that why I'm so sore after exercising?

The pain you're feeling is acute inflammation. It results from the tiny tears that exercise causes in your muscles.

If you are sore, take a day off. As you rest, your body will repair the tears, and in the process make your

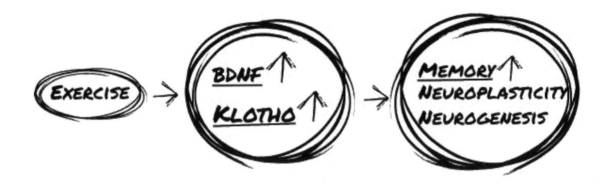

The benefits of exercise for the brain

muscles stronger. Ultimately, when you exercise, chronic inflammation throughout your body will decrease.

Two Proteins that Increase with Exercise

Brain-derived neurotrophic factor (BDNF)

For many years, we believed that there was no coming back from the cellular loss that results from brain trauma, toxins and other sources of neuroinflammation. Once gone, gone forever.

This is not true.

We now realize that our neurons have potential for recovery, repair and regeneration thanks to a protein in your brain called *brain-derived neurotrophic factor,* or BDNF.

BDNF has the power to replace lost neurons with new ones and heal damaged cells.[29] Think of BDNF as "Miracle-Gro" for the brain.[30]

Many researchers have associated low levels of BDNF with Alzheimer's disease, depression, memory loss and other cognitive problems. Increasing your BDNF is an excellent way to reduce your risk of Alzheimer's disease.

The best way to increase BDNF is to exercise, especially aerobic exercise or high-intensity interval workouts have proven effective. (More on these later.)

Klotho

Klotho is another essential protein that increases with regular exercise. According to Dena Dubal, klotho "acts to make tighter, better connections at the synapse."[31] These help to optimize many functions of the brain.

Klotho has become known for its anti-aging properties because it can have such a significant effect on IQ, memory and muscle regeneration. Scientists now think it may be able to improve our ability to learn and remember.[32]

But don't expect to take a pill to increase your klotho anytime soon. The research is too new. For now, the best way we know to increase klotho is steady aerobic exercise sustained over 12 weeks.[33]

Exercise That Benefits the Brain

Aerobic Exercise

Aerobic exercise includes brisk walking, swimming, cycling and any other exercise that increases your heart rate. You need to start slow and work your way up to a healthy level of physical training. Start with five minutes a day and keep adding time as you can until you reach 30 minutes, five days a week.

In addition to helping the heart deliver healthy nutrients to your brain, aerobic exercise is also thought to improve *neuronal plasticity*—which means your brain's ability to adapt to changes. Aerobic exercise also increases choline in the brain, which may prevent further cognitive decline.[34]

For all these reasons, aerobic exercise is one of the best lifestyle choices you can make for your cognitive health.

High-Intensity Interval Training

Interval training involves alternating between fast (high-intensity) and slow (low-intensity) exercise. You are at the top end of your power only for short periods—15, 30, 45 or 60 seconds—before returning to low or moderate intensity.

A research team at Mayo Clinic found that high-intensity interval training slows aging at the cellular level. This is probably because interval training increases your BDNF, important for your cells.[35]

Strength training

Strength and resistance training uses weights to improve muscle strength. This training enhances cognitive performance and brain function, especially problem-solving. Strength training also helps you manage your body weight, boost your metabolism and increase bone density.

After checking with your doctor, choose a free weight that causes you to tire after lifting it 12 to 15 times.[36] Increase your repetitions from there, but remember to take at least a day off between sessions if you become sore.

Flexibility and Balance

Flexibility and balance exercises will help prevent falls as you age, and that's enormously important for the brain. These exercises require many interconnected and multisensory thoughts so as you do them you are giving your brain a "cognitive workout" as well. In order to balance, you have to use sight, your inner ear, joint receptors and your muscles, and all those instructions go through the brain. You can find simple flexibility and balance exercises online. Remember, it's important to have a "spotter" nearby to help with balance if you need it.[37]

Tips for Your Exercise Plan

Before you start, please see your doctor. Your doctor can do a complete review of your health and your risks before clearing you for physical activity and movement.

Manage acute inflammation: Take a day off after intense exercise so that your muscles have a chance to heal.

Don't stop: If you stop exercising, then you stop receiving any anti-aging, anti-cancer, anti-disease and anti-Alzheimer's benefits. Exercise is a lifelong prescription.

How to Maintain Your Motivation

- *Track your progress:* This will help keep you motivated.

- *Exercise with a friend or a family member*: This helps to keep you accountable.

- If you can, *hire a personal trainer or wellness coach*.

- *Stick with your exercise*: Make sure it's not too hard and that it fits your lifestyle. You'll know it's working when you start looking forward to exercising regularly.

- *It's not all or nothing:* Life happens. If you get away from exercise for a week or so, don't use that as an excuse to stop completely. Again, regular exercise is a lifetime prescription!

One more suggestion: Consider going outside

The best exercise plan is the one you enjoy enough to keep doing. Lifting weights, stretching and walking on a treadmill are all good, but you may find that going outside, especially with a friend or loved one, is even better.

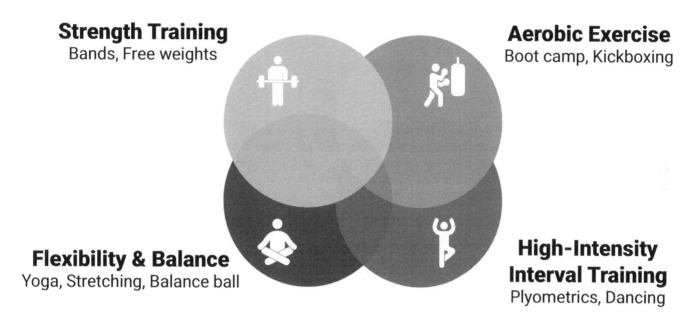

Strength Training
Bands, Free weights

Aerobic Exercise
Boot camp, Kickboxing

Flexibility & Balance
Yoga, Stretching, Balance ball

**High-Intensity
Interval Training**
Plyometrics, Dancing

Four kinds of exercise that offer special benefits to your brain.

There's always something to enjoy outside whether it's cold, warm, windy, cloudy or sunny. The "outdoor experience" adds to your physical exercise by stimulating and saturating all your senses. You can breathe deeply, enjoy the scenery and listen to the sounds of nature. You might even try going barefoot so you can feel the earth under your feet.

Believe me: You'll find it incredibly refreshing!

Chapter 7
Rid Your Body of Increased Oxidation

Don't let your brain and body become rusty.

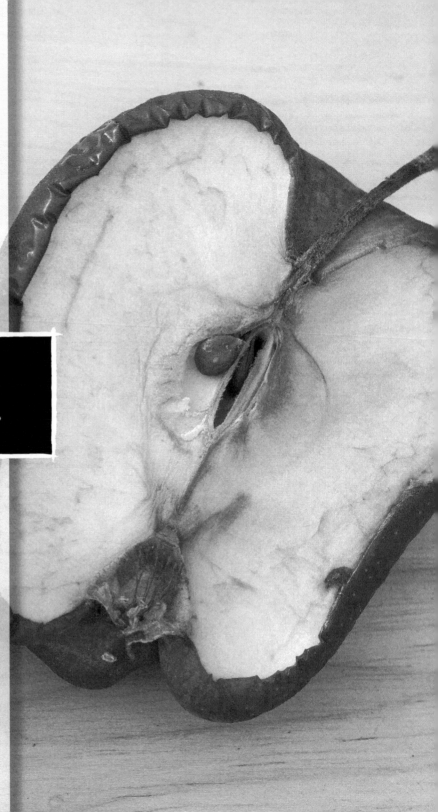

In this chapter, I want to explain *oxidation*, a process that is very damaging to the cells in your whole body and, of course, your brain.

You've almost certainly seen oxidation. It's the brown that develops when you leave a half-eaten apple on the counter or when a car rusts. You can also see its effects in the thin, wrinkly skin of elderly people.

Over time, oxidation decreases the number of healthy cells in your body to devastating effect, especially in your brain.

What Happens in Oxidation?

Whether in an apple, a car, an older adult's skin or your brain, oxidation occurs when an instigating molecule robs an electron from another nearby atom. This theft destabilizes the diminished atom or molecule, making it a free radical.

People in a radical political movement have often lost something—a job, their home, their family. Without them, radicals seem to lose their mooring and may even become violent lawbreakers.

In the same way, a free radical in your body has also lost something—the electron that the instigating molecule stole. To replace that electron, the free radical steals an electron from another nearby atom. That theft starts a frenzied chain reaction. More and more molecules lose electrons and then steal from other atoms, resulting in an explosion of damage.

Often the cells and tissues where this is happening can't keep up with all the damage and your immune system joins the fight.

When this happens, chronic inflammation occurs, and this adds to the cellular damage. Soon your body systems begin to suffer as well.

You have experienced this system damage if you have diabetes, depression, heart trouble, lung disease or other chronic conditions. All these conditions began in your cells, at least partially because of oxidation. In your 60s or 70s, you'll probably see this "rusting" in your skin as well.

Alzheimer's is one of these chronic diseases, so if you want to avoid Alzheimer's, limiting oxidation in your body is an important step.

What Causes Oxidation?

These disruptive molecules come from the environment around you, including air and water pollution, cleaning supplies and pesticides. Others come from food, stress and lack of sleep. To limit the possibility of free radicals, avoid the following:

- *Hazardous environmental toxins*: These include cigarette smoke, toxic metals, air pollution, pesticides, radiation and industrial chemicals.
- *Refined sugars.* (See Chapter 9.)
- *Alcohol in excess.*
- *Vegetable oils exposed to heat and light.* Most are high in Omega-6 fatty acids. They encourage oxidation. Also, oil heated past its "smoke point" produces free radicals. Reused oil is one reason fast food is so dangerous to your health.
- *Processed meats*: The fat in processed meats produces free radicals over high heat.

How to Limit Oxidation

To review, free radicals cause damage by stealing electrons from other atoms. If your body had no defense against this process, we would probably all die young!

Fortunately, some atoms have an electron to spare. They can donate one of their electrons to the rampaging free radical and still remain stable. When

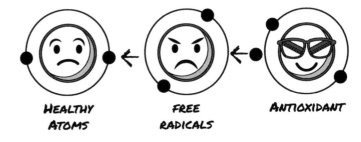

HEALTHY ATOMS   FREE RADICALS   ANTIOXIDANT

Free radical scavengers

this happens, the destructive chain reaction stops in its tracks.

Peace!

These generous atoms are called ***antioxidants***. They enter a volatile situation and provide a compromise that defuses the violence.

Phytonutrients in plant-based foods provide some of the best antioxidants. These natural chemicals protect plants and keep them healthy. They can do the same for you. You'll learn more about them in Chapter 10.

Here are foods and drinks that will slow down oxidation in your body:

- Blueberries (always high on lists of antioxidants)
- Red berries like raspberries and strawberries
- Dark-colored (purple or red) grapes
- Oranges, chili peppers, lemons, limes and other foods high in Vitamin C
- Fish that are rich in omega-3, such as salmon, trout and sardines
- Nuts, especially walnuts and Brazil nuts

- Dark green veggies—especially broccoli, spinach, kale and collard greens
- Sweet potatoes and orange vegetables, like carrots and butternut and acorn squash
- Whole grains—switching from white bread to whole grain bread will help
- Beans—black beans, kidney beans, lentils, soybeans and black-eyed peas
- Tea, especially green tea
- Foods like apples, onions, cranberries, dark chocolate and red wine that are high in *flavonoids* (a kind of phytonutrient)

In this book, I will be stressing how important fruits and vegetables are to your health. Their effect on oxidation is a first reason to make them a bigger part of your daily eating.

The Question of Supplements

If you do take supplements, be sure to talk to your doctor first. Always take the recommended daily amount because higher doses could increase oxidation.

Also, it's always better to get nutrients from food. Instead of supplements, you could increase the following foods in your diet:

- *Beta-carotene:* in carrots, sweet potatoes, spinach and kale, cantaloupe and apricots
- *Lutein:* in kale, winter squash, collard greens, spinach and chard
- *Lycopene:* in tomatoes, watermelon, purple cabbage, carrots and mangoes
- *Selenium:* in eggs, mushrooms, oats, Brazil nuts and many kinds of meat
- *Vitamin A:* in cooked sweet potato, cooked winter squash, cooked kale, carrots, sweet bell peppers, meat and liver
- *Vitamin C:* in strawberries, pineapple, kohlrabi, mangoes, Brussels sprouts, kiwi, bell peppers, oranges and broccoli
- *Vitamin E:* in almonds, Swiss chard, mustard greens, spinach and kale, avocado, broccoli, olives and plant oils

What Does All This Mean for Your Brain?

Let's say a toxin with free radicals crosses your blood-brain barrier. These free radicals begin stealing electrons from cells in your brain, and a destructive chain reaction results.

If you have introduced enough antioxidants into your body through healthy nutrients, these antioxidants will be available to halt the chain reaction, calm the inflammation that developed as a result of oxidation and preserve the health of your brain cells.

Your entire body will feel better and your risk of Alzheimer's will decrease.

Chapter 8

Rid Your Body of Threats to Your Mitochondria

For your memory, optimizing your cell engine is half of the answer.

Tiny structures in your cells called *mitochondria* produce the energy that your body needs. Think of them as the engines that keep your body running.[38]

First, your blood delivers nutrients and oxygen to the cell and eventually enters your cell's mitochondria. Some human cells have up to 10,000 of these little engines.

Mitochondria do their thing and then release high-energy molecules called ATP into the cell. ATP passes this energy to another molecule in the cell, which now has the energy it needs to function.

If you have a faulty engine in your car, it won't work. In the same way, if you have faulty mitochondria, your cells won't work. Functioning mitochondria are crucial to your overall health and especially to the health of your brain.

The brain has 100 billion cells called neurons (give or take a few billion) and about one trillion synapses (the connecting points between neurons). Transmitting electrical charges through so many neurons and across so many synapses requires a *lot* of energy.

In fact, your brain uses 20% of your body's energy even though your brain is only 2% of your body by weight. Its constant need for energy makes your brain very sensitive to any damage to your mitochondria.

In this chapter, I will explain how you can help keep your mitochondria healthy so your brain functions well.

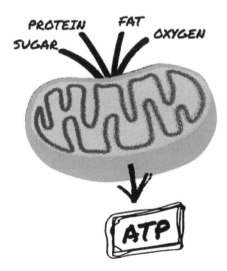

Mitochondria produce energy for your cells.

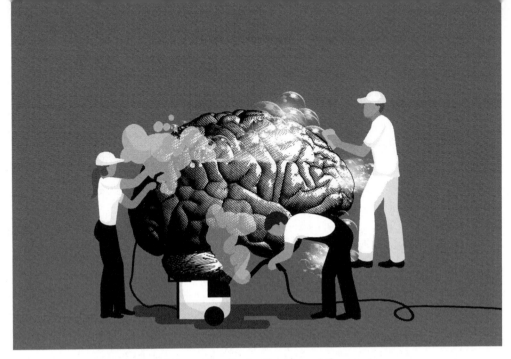

Mitochondria refresh the brain with new energy.

Oxidation, the Greatest Threat

During the process of mitochondria producing energy, there's a great deal of potential for damage from oxidation.

1. First, when mitochondria transfer ATP to other molecules, they sometimes drop an unpaired electron, also known as a free radical. (See Chapter 7.) These free radicals cause an explosion of inflammatory damage inside the cell, which can often lead to cell death.

2. Second, the energy from mitochondria can fuel the inflammation, making it even more explosive—like stored gasoline adding to the explosiveness of a gas station fire.

3. Third, because every cell in your body has not one but many mitochondria, the chronic inflammation that results from free radicals can occur anytime and anywhere in your body.

In the brain, the mitochondria damaged by free radicals can harm your neurons, which you may remember carry messages in your brain.[39] These damaged neurons contribute to weakness and pain in your extremities as well as problems in your brain.

Your glial cells, the bodyguards and janitors of your neurons, also suffer. They become unable to remove toxins from the nervous system. As these toxins accumulate, they cause memory impairment, brain fog, and additional inflammation. Eventually, a full range of diseases in the brain can result, including Alzheimer's.

Fortunately, antioxidants can stop the explosive process of oxidation and inflammation that occurs around mitochondria. So give your body lots of the antioxidant foods listed in Chapter 7.

Other Hazards to Mitochondria

- **Poor Nutrition:** You need high-quality nutrients for your mitochondria to work well. If you think of mitochondria as engines, unhealthy foods are like poor-quality gasoline that ruins the car's efficiency and may even damage the car.

- **Inactivity:** Physical activity improves your circulation and oxygenation, enhancing mitochondrial function. High-intensity interval training will increase brain-derived neurotrophic factor, which increases the quantity and quality of your brain's mitochondria.

- **Air Pollution:** Mitochondria use oxygen to produce energy, so good quality air is the power that drives the mitochondrial factory. Sources of low-quality air include smoking, smog, car exhaust and burning leaves, so take steps to protect your mitochondria from these contaminants. (See Chapter 19.)

- **Environmental Toxins:** These include heavy metals, pesticides and herbicides, which also contribute to mitochondrial damage. (See Chapter 19.)

- **Lack of Iron in Your Blood:** If you get too much iron, that's a problem, but if your diet lacks sufficient iron, you won't have enough hemoglobin to carry oxygen. The deficiency puts pressure on your heart and lungs and indirectly hurts your mitochondria. Talk to your doctor about ways to increase your iron levels if you think they might be low.

- **Unnecessary or Overuse of Medications:** Overmedicating causes widespread problems in your body, so be careful about taking medications you don't need.

There's Hope!

The brain has incredible recovery and rehabilitative abilities. As you work on modifiable lifestyle factors like sleep, nutrition, toxins and others, your mitochondria will respond.

An active and stimulating life filled with healthy choices will improve the quantity and quality of your mitochondria and bring new energy to your life.

Chapter 9
Rid Your Body of Refined Sugar

Sweet in your mouth, sour in your brain.

In the next chapter, on nutrition, I explain how to choose the most healthy carbohydrates to eat. So why have I dedicated an entire chapter to sugar?

Because of all the things you put in your mouth, refined sugar is one of the most damaging to your health and cognitive abilities.

By refined sugar, I mean sugar that has been removed from its natural sources, purified and then turned into a form that we can add to other foods. It might help to think of it as "added sugar."

In July 2018, the Federal Food and Drug Administration began requiring that most packaged foods add this term to their food labels. The FDA wanted to make it easier for consumers to know the amount of refined sugar each product contained.

Sources for refined sugars include cane sugar, sugar beets and corn. Manufacturers process these sugars into granulated sugar, powdered sugar, high fructose corn syrup, brown sugar, molasses, coconut palm sugar, agave, straight glucose or any other form they can dream up.

No matter what you call these refined sugars, they are all bad for you! Once removed from their natural sources, none of them has any nutritive value.[40] As for energy, refined sugars usually add to your fatigue.

Naturally occurring sugars in fruits, vegetables and other foods come packaged with fiber, vitamins, antioxidants and other healthy nutrients. All these extras—especially the fiber in fruits and vegetables—slow the absorption of sugar into the blood, protecting you from sugar spikes.

A sugar spike is a sudden infusion of sugar into your bloodstream. The less fiber attached to the sugar (think soft drinks and candy), the higher the sugar spike.

After my death scare, one early change I made was to remove refined sugar and artificial sweeteners from my diet. I had become quite addicted to Cinnamon Toast Crunch cereal and sweetened yogurt. How unhealthy could those be? Then I totaled the amount of refined sugar I was eating every day: between 10 and 14 tablespoons (almost a cup) of sugar each day, depending on how many bowls of cereal I ate.

The recommended amount of refined sugar for men is only 3 tablespoons. This means I was getting three or four times that daily from just those two foods!

The average American consumes 7 tablespoons per day, 6 cups a week, or 312 cups a year.[41] Refined, or added, sugar accounts for about 500 calories each day in the average American diet, with a third of those calories coming from sugary soft drinks.

Unfortunately, refined sugar is added to many processed foods. You'll have a hard time finding any food in the grocery store, outside the produce and meat sections, that does *not* have added sugar.

Nothing healthy comes from all this refined sugar, not for your body and definitely not for your brain.

The Damage Sugar Spikes Cause

As mentioned, in the absence of fiber, your body converts refined sugar into glucose very quickly, causing that sugar spike in your bloodstream. Unless you have diabetes, your body can usually adjust to this spike.

Not so your brain. Every sudden infusion of sugar harms your brain, whether you have diabetes or not.

The brain needs a steady source of glucose to function properly. Any extreme infusion of sugar into the brain is dangerous for both diabetics and nondiabetics.

Your brain reacts to sugar spikes with an immune response that can lead to chronic inflammation. Scientists offer four reasons why the brain reacts so strongly to sugar spikes.

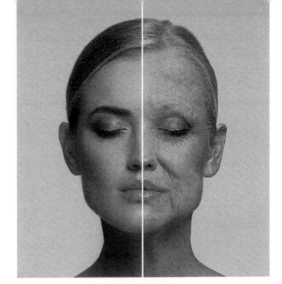

The effects of glycation

1. Damage to blood vessels from glycation

Glycation occurs when too much sugar enters your system all at once. The excessive sugar bonds with proteins, creating toxic compounds called *advanced glycation end products*, or AGEs. These AGEs keep the proteins from doing their work.

If sustained, glycation causes your blood vessels throughout your body to tighten. Glycation also leads to cataracts, wrinkled skin and other problems associated with aging.

It's true. ***Too much sugar makes you look older.***[42]

Glycation can stiffen blood vessels in the brain and make blood flow difficult. The stiffened blood vessels have trouble delivering nutrients, and that means the brain gets less energy than it needs.

"The more the arteries become damaged," nutrition expert Patrick Holford says, "the worse the circulation to the brain and the less reliable the supply of nutrients becomes. So, ironically, eating too much sugar can lead to temporary glucose starvation to cells."[43]

The brain sees glycation-damaged proteins as a threat, so microglia rush to where they are, causing neuroinflammation. Short-term, the microglia can deal with the threat, but if you repeatedly cause sugar spikes—*whether or not you have diabetes*—the neuroinflammation becomes chronic, and your brain suffers.

No wonder I experienced "brain fog" during the days I was eating so much Cinnamon Toast Crunch.

2. Macrophage migration inhibitory factor damage

Sugar spikes in the brain also damage an enzyme called the macrophage migration inhibitory factor (MIF).[44] Undamaged MIF helps the immune cells protect the brain from abnormal proteins. When sugar damages the MIF, the immune cells go into overdrive, causing too much inflammation. This increases your risk of Alzheimer's.

3. Impaired BNDF

Sugar spikes are the enemy of brain-derived neurotrophic factor (BDNF), the chemical in the brain that helps maintain neurons and create new ones. BDNF also:

- Protects your ability to form new memories and to learn and remember

- Protects against the damage that stress does to your brain cells

- Helps your neural pathways—the communication highway for your brain—to stay supple and active

4. Explosive free radicals in the brain

In the brain, sugar spikes "sugar-coat" proteins so they release an excessive number of free radicals. Glycation-damaged proteins, for example, produce 50 times more free radicals than other proteins.[45]

Your brain correctly perceives these sugar-damaged proteins as a threat, so it rushes microglia to the scene to fight the process. If sugar spikes keep coming throughout your day, the microglia cannot keep up and chronic neuroinflammation results.

Pay attention the next time you eat too many sweets. Doesn't your brain begin to feel foggy?

We still have more to learn about the effect of sugar spikes on the brain, but for now, if you want to keep your brain healthy, limit your intake of added sugar.

Diabetes, A Deadly Threat to the Brain

I've already said glycation hinders the ability of blood vessels to deliver nutrients throughout the brain. Because your brain needs so much energy compared to the rest of your body, diabetes is an even greater threat to your brain.

Diabetes, in all its forms, involves problems with insulin, a hormone that regulates how much sugar is in your blood. Insulin is important because it helps to move sugar out of the blood into cells where they can use it for energy. With diabetes, either because the body stops producing insulin or the body stops responding to insulin, the sugar has trouble reaching the cells.[46]

How a Healthy Body Processes Sugar

1. A healthy person eats something with carbohydrates in it. Carbohydrates have sugar.

2. The carbohydrates are broken down into single units of sugar. If the carbohydrates have fiber, that slows the process so that the body does not experience a sugar spike.

3. Sugar (mostly glucose) from the carbohydrates goes into the bloodstream.

4. An insulin-signaling system moves sugar from the blood into the cells.

5. Once sugar enters the cells, it is converted into energy.

6. If no cells need energy, insulin helps move the extra sugar out of the bloodstream into the liver and muscles for storage. (Once the liver and muscles can't hold any more sugar, excess is stored as fat.)

Kinds of Diabetes (see chart)

The immune system of people with Type I diabetes destroys insulin. They have to take insulin every day.

People with Type 2 diabetes produce insulin, but the body resists its effect, so too much sugar stays in the blood.

This disease is caused by too much sugar in the diet, coupled with other factors like obesity, physical inactivity and family history.

Diabetes doubles your risk of Alzheimer's dementia,[47] so avoiding or managing this disease is vitally important.

Dr. Vera Novak, a professor of neurology at Harvard Medical School, and her colleagues studied a group of 65 senior adults, about half with Type 2 diabetes and the rest without it. In just two years, those with diabetes were scoring lower on cognitive tests than they had at the beginning of the study. Those without diabetes showed no change.[48]

A Brain-Specific Diabetes

As I said, an extremely complex insulin-signaling system is necessary to move sugar out of the blood into cells. Based on studies of deceased patients' brain tissue, scientists are fairly certain that, with Alzheimer's, the insulin-signalling system in the brain fails. This causes neurons to starve for energy and die.

Because this insulin resistance is so specific to the brain, many experts now consider Alzheimer's

The Three Types of Diabetes				
Type	**Where insulin comes from**	**How it operates**	**Cause**	**Treatment**
Type 1 diabetes	Pancreas	The immune system destroys insulin-producing cells in the pancreas	Strong genetic component	Daily insulin
Type 2 diabetes	Pancreas	Cells cannot identify or absorb insulin released by the pancreas, so sugar tends to stay in the blood	Obesity and/or a family history of diabetes	Weight loss, healthy eating, exercise, lifestyle changes, medication (sometimes insulin)
Type 3 diabetes	Brain	The insulin-signaling-system in the brain becomes ineffective so sugar cannot get out of the bloodstream into neurons. This leads to cell damage and possibly to Alzheimer's.	Associated with Type 2 diabetes, but the actual cause is unknown and remains the subject of research	Scientists are researching possible treatments for Alzheimer's using diabetes medications

dementia Type III diabetes. Scientists are exploring the possibility of treating Alzheimer's with diabetes medication.[49] In the meantime, it's best to avoid overtaxing your brain with too much sugar.

How to Cut Down on Sugar in Your Diet

Let's be honest: Sugar tastes good. Our first natural food—mother's milk—is quite sweet.[50] From an early age, we've been programmed to like sweetness. But if you want your brain to be healthy, you need to cut down or eliminate refined sugar from your diet.

Given how pervasive refined sugar is in the Standard American Diet (SAD), how good it tastes and its nostalgic associations with so many of our holidays, how can we possibly limit or remove it from our diets?

The following page lists many suggestions.

1. **Eliminate drinks with either sugar or artificial sweeteners.**

   - Begin with one less drink a day and work your way down to none
   - Experiment with adding slices of lemon, lime or fresh mint to water
   - Try green tea, which has the added benefit of being high in antioxidants
   - Try other teas, including herbal teas, either hot or iced

2. **Eliminate sweets during the day.** Do donuts often appear at your office? Have an alternative treat ready at your desk: fruit, nuts or roasted chickpeas. One of my favorite snacks is dried mulberries—naturally low in sugar and high in fiber and antioxidants.

3. **During the week, have fruit for dessert.** You may have to retrain your taste buds, but you can do it!

   - Start with one or two evenings per week, and go up from there.
   - Begin with fruits you particularly like and expand gradually.
   - Eat fresh fruit that's in season (it will taste better).
   - Bit by bit, the thought of eating fruit will become more appealing.

4. **Continue to enjoy an occasional sweet treat,** maybe once on the weekend or at a special party. Once you start limiting sugar, you may find that you crave it less. As time goes on, make added sugar an increasingly rare indulgence—a bite or two of rich desserts at anniversaries and birthdays. However, if you are particularly susceptible to sugar cravings, you may have to cut refined sugar out of your diet completely.

5. **Don't skimp on proteins and healthy fats.** These will keep you full longer. Vegetable-based protein from beans and legumes have the added advantage of giving you lots of fiber, keeping you full even longer.

6. **Avoid sugar substitutes.** More on that later.

7. **"Process" your foods at home.** In other words, make your sauces, salad dressings, smoothies and other foods yourself. Then you'll know how much refined sugar goes into each of them.

8. **If you do buy processed foods, read food labels.** A quick survey of bottled marinara sauce, for instance, shows that ½ cup can have as many as 12 g of sugar or as few as 1 g (with zero added sugar). Of course, added sugar is only one ingredient to consider—the kind of fat also matters—but always keep sugar in mind when you purchase prepared foods.

   Here are some names of hidden sugars: corn sweetener, corn syrup, maltose, sucrose, high-fructose corn syrup, dextrose, evaporated cane juice, malt syrup, lactose and fruit juice concentrates.[51]

Other Ways to Control Blood Sugar

1. **Exercise**: Aerobic exercise (like brisk walking) combined with resistance training limits insulin resistance. Start slow, keep going and pretty soon you'll be surprised how much better you feel.

2. **Limit unhealthy fats:** They accumulate in the bloodstream, hindering the work of insulin. The effect of these fats is almost immediate. Eat a meal with unhealthy fat, and within three hours, your insulin resistance will increase.[52] Eliminate unhealthy fat, and your insulin will begin to work better. Sources of unhealthy fats include trans fats, palm oil and margarine. Excessive consumption of saturated fats found in meat, dairy and coconut is harmful.[53] In the United States, the #1 source of saturated fat is pizza.[54]

3. **Lose weight:** A better diet coupled with exercise will help you lose weight. Weighing less will lower your blood sugar and have a positive effect on your insulin levels.

What About Artificial Sweeteners?

Before closing this chapter, I want to say a few words about artificial sweeteners. I recommend that you avoid them entirely. I don't think they are safe.

In the interest of transparency, however, I must admit that not everyone agrees with me. Research is ongoing, but why take the risk?

As for weight loss or blood sugar control, there is no evidence that artificial sugars help these efforts. Quite the opposite. A ten-year study published by the *Canadian Medical Association Journal* indicated that people who consumed them were actually at high risk for weight gain, diabetes and heart disease.

Many researchers believe sweeteners trick your mind into thinking real sweetness is on its way. Your brain then prompts you to seek out real sugar, and you end up eating too much of the wrong foods. The Harvard Medical School has published an excellent critique of artificial sweeteners.[55]

We do not know what long-term use of artificial sweeteners will do to our health, but I suspect it's not good. Far better to enjoy the natural sweetness of fruits.

The Bottom Line

Refined, or added, sugar should not be part of your regular diet. Reserve it for special occasions—or refuse to touch it at all.

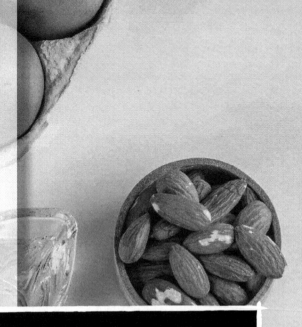

Chapter 10

Rid Your Body of Nutritional Problems

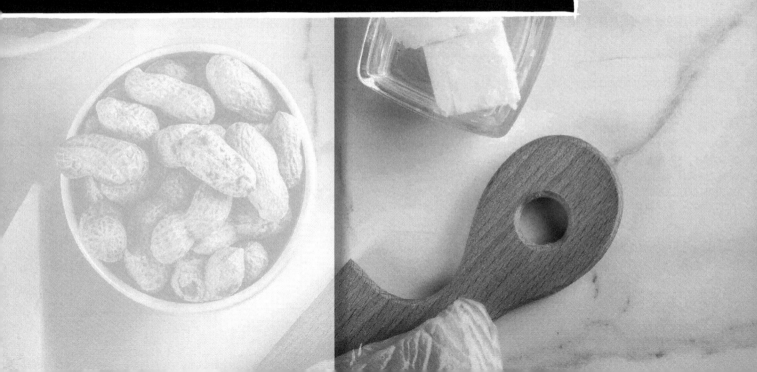

> *"Our food should be our medicine and our medicine should be our food."*
>
> — Hippocrates

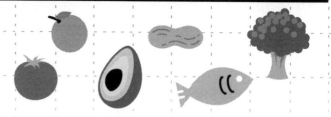

FIGHT INFLAMMATION

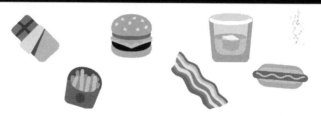

CAUSE INFLAMMATION

Anti-inflammatory vs. inflammatory foods

Day by day, the food and drink you introduce into your body affects your health.

In this section, I will provide a platform of nutritional information that will help you reduce your risk of Alzheimer's dementia. If it all seems a little intimidating, please remember that healthy eating is a lifetime journey. Better nutrition each day leads to a better tomorrow.

Anti-Inflammatory Foods

Throughout this nutritional platform, I will stress foods that decrease your inflammation. The wrong food choices can trigger inflammation throughout your body.

We've already discussed sugar. The wrong fats can do the same, as can processed meats, soda (diet or regular), fast foods and other foods that are staples of the Standard American Diet (SAD).

Your body uses inflammation to try to deal with these bad food choices. The immune cells involved with inflammation end up damaging and even killing cells throughout your body.

Because inflammation is so hard on your brain, the nutritional platform I describe includes many weapons against inflammation.

Is This a New Diet I Should Follow?

Last time I checked different diets available online, I saw more than 93 different diets—detox diets, diabetic diets, blood-pressure-lowering diets, low-fat and high-fat diets (ketogenic), vegetarian and vegan diets, gluten-free and dozens more.

Because you are unique, I will not be proposing a new diet. For this to work, you will need to make choices that fit your lifestyle, family preferences, interests and health needs.

What I offer instead is a viewpoint that will improve your overall health. As you look through this chapter, please remember:

- Nothing I say here is new. It is, instead, based on a proven personal journey.

- The subject of this book is not weight loss. If you choose to follow up on this information, you may find yourself losing weight, but weight loss is not the primary intention.

- This chapter does not stand alone. It works alongside many of the other modifiable lifestyle factors described in this book to lower your risk of Alzheimer's.

Keeping Things in Balance

I'm also not suggesting that you give up all pleasures in your life related to food and drink—unless that is something you want.

Well-known Food Network chef Alton Brown famously gave up fast food when he decided to improve his health, and as far as I know, he's holding to that decision. If you want to add some "don'ts" to your nutritional platform, go for it.

Most of us, however, succeed with a more moderate approach—one without any "don'ts." I suggest you think of your diet in terms of three concentric rings.

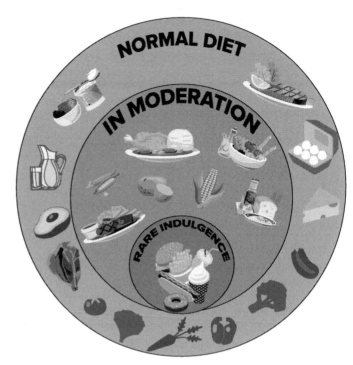

A Moderate Approach to Food Choices

1. ***Most of the time:*** The biggest ring is for what you typically eat—good-for-you, healthy food.

2. ***Occasionally:*** A smaller ring is for what you eat in moderation—pasta, fried rice or steak on a date with your spouse.

3. ***Rarely:*** The third, *very* small ring is for more rare indulgences (cake at your daughter's wedding, Chinese food to celebrate your son's graduation, ribs on your own birthday).

This way you don't have to think of a future where you can never enjoy a chocolate chip cookie!

A Healthy Nutritional Platform

The following nutritional platform will help your brain and nervous system work better.

It depends primarily on pesticide-free, plant-based nutrients, the right kind of fats and hormone-free protein.

Plant-Based Nutrients

The cornerstone of your diet should be the nutrients found in plants. These include any foods that come directly from a plant.

Eating more fruits, vegetables and other plant-based foods is good for your overall health and will definitely help your brain and nervous system work better.

Plant-based nutrients decrease your risk for many chronic illnesses. They also help you see, smell, taste, hear, walk, learn and think better, and improve your balance, mood and emotional health.

Scientists, physicians and nutrition experts generally agree that more fruits and vegetables will improve your health. This is one nutritional change you can make with complete confidence.

Benefits of Fruits and Vegetables

Fiber

We need fiber for regular bowel movements, a healthy gut, better cholesterol and healthy blood sugar levels. Fiber also helps us maintain a healthy weight.

The fiber in your diet comes exclusively from plant sources. Animals have bones to hold them up; plants have fiber, so if you need to increase the fiber in your diet, eat more plant-based foods, including:

- Whole grains
- Vegetables
- Beans, peas and other legumes
- Fruits
- Nuts and seeds

Remember, the more processed or refined your foods, the less fiber you receive from them. Opt for whole foods: an orange rather than juice; fresh peaches rather than canned; oat groats or oat bran rather than cold oat cereal.

Vitamins and Minerals

Fruits, vegetables and other plant-based whole foods are rich in vitamins, which are essential for health. (See Chapter 12.)

Antioxidants

Antioxidants, remember, are foods with atoms that fight oxidation. They have an electron to spare that they can share with atoms or molecules that have had an electron stolen. (See Chapter 7.)

Most of the highest-ranked antioxidant sources come from fruits and vegetables.

Phytonutrients

These nutrients, present in beautiful and colorful plants, are the cheapest and most powerful medicine known to human beings. You may recognize these: beta-carotene (found in carrots), lycopene (in tomatoes) and resveratrol (in dark red and purple grapes). There are many more.

In plants, these nutrients guard against insects, pollution and disease. They can protect your body as well.

Phytonutrients are especially powerful anti-inflammatory agents. They deliver a lot of antioxidants to your body—on average 64 times more than animal foods.[56] In reducing your risk of Alzheimer's, you can't go wrong eating fruits and vegetables!

How can you know that you are getting a variety of these phytonutrients? It's easy! Eat fruits and vegetables of many different colors. See the chart on the next page.

How to Create a Plant-Based Eating Plan

Remember, I'm not advocating a completely vegetarian or vegan eating plan. I'm just encouraging you to have plant-based foods fill more of your plate and keep meat and other animal-based products like cheese and cream—if you really want them—as a condiment or side dish.

1. **Plan:** So often unhealthy foods result from rushing our choices. Fast food on the way home from work, ordering in a quick sandwich at your desk for lunch or pizza in the evening. Homemade, plant-based foods can be almost as simple and convenient if you plan ahead.

2. **Find healthy recipes that satisfy:** Follow food blogs that have recipes for fruits and vegetables. Check out cookbooks from the library. Ask for great recipes on Facebook. And when you find a recipe for fruits and vegetables that you like, keep it handy.

3. **Start with breakfast:** Choose whole grain toast with nut butter or avocado, whole grain tortillas wrapped around a mix of vegetables or a bowl of oatmeal (use fruit to sweeten, not sugar).

4. **Correct your lunch choices:** Salads, soups or nourishing smoothies are great options, along with wraps with lots of fresh veggies.

5. **Revise snacks:** Along with whole fruits and vegetables, snack on unsalted or lightly salted nuts.

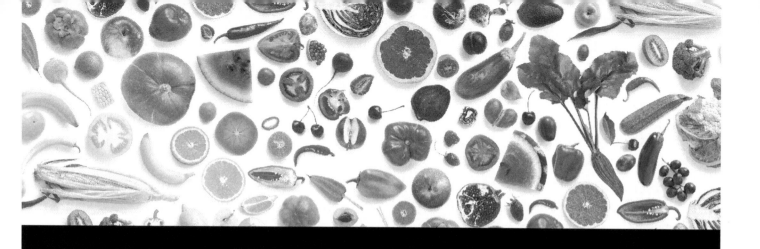

ORANGE

apricots, cantaloupes, carrots, mangos, bell peppers, nectarines, oranges, papayas, pumpkins, squash, sweet potatoes, tangerines, yams, turmeric roots (turmeric). They are rich in Vitamin C, protect against infection, boost the immune system, make skin healthy, help breathing and keep the blood supply healthy.
PHYTONUTRIENTS: beta-carotene, cryptoxanthin, herperidin, citrus bioflavonoids.

GREEN

asparagus, avocados, bell peppers, broccoli, Brussels sprouts, cabbage, cucumbers, olives, zucchini; rich potassium, vitamin C, vitamin K, and folic acid. They help balance hormones, detoxify the body, boost the immune system, and prevent cancer. These foods are excellent for your brain and heart and allow you to live a longer and healthier life.
PHYTONUTRIENTS: chlorophyll, lutein/zeaxanthin, EGCG, isoflavones, sulphoraphane.

WHITE

cauliflower, coconuts, dates, garlic, ginger, chickpeas, lentils, mushrooms, nuts, onions, pears, seeds, rice, grains, tea, coffee.

PURPLE

grapes, blueberries, blackberries, bell peppers, cabbage, carrots, cauliflower, eggplants, figs, kale, olives, prunes, rice (black or purple). They are anti-inflammatory, anti-cancer, antioxidant compounds that help protect the brain and heart, improve blood sugar levels and cholesterol and limit thyroid problems.
PHYTOCHEMICALS: resveratrol, proanthocyanidins, bioflavonoids.

YELLOW

lemons, ginger roots, bell peppers, bananas, apples, pineapples, succotash, squash. They are good sources of vitamin C or A.
PHYTONUTRIENTS: lutein/zeaxanthin

Eat a rainbow of fruits and vegetables!

6. **Now for the hardest part, your evening meals:** At dinner, fill 2/3 of your plate with vegetables and eat fruit for dessert on most evenings.

7. **When you do eat out:** Look first at the salads, sides and soups because they generally include more vegetables.

8. **Indulge intentionally:** Remember, this new platform involves changing your everyday eating habits. Special days still deserve celebrations. Just remember to return to healthy patterns.

Good Fats Help the Brain (Oil up, America!)

Your brain is 60% fat, so you need a plentiful supply of healthy fats to reduce your risk of Alzheimer's.

How much is enough?

I recommend you proportion your daily calories as follows: 50-60% of your calories from fats, 20-25% from proteins, and 20-25% from carbohydrates—and these mostly from fruits and vegetables.

That may seem like a lot of fat, but remember, fat is calorie dense, meaning that fat packs a lot of calories into minimal volume.

- A cup of broccoli has 31 calories.
- A cup of lean ground chicken has 300.

- A cup of olive oil has 1,908 calories.

The volume of fruits, vegetables and lean protein add up quickly compared to fats. For every two tablespoons of olive oil (238 calories), you would need to eat eight cups of broccoli!

I'm not recommending that you eat unlimited amounts of fats, even "good" ones. Too much fat will increase your risk of cardiovascular disease, diabetes, along with a host of other chronic problems, including Alzheimer's.

I'm just suggesting that you are intentional about getting enough fat.

How Too Little Fat Affects Your Body

For years, we were bombarded with advice to maintain a very low-fat diet, but that advice is under scrutiny. Many scientists now believe that inadequate fat in your diet can have dire consequences, especially for your brain:

- If you often feel hungry, fat can keep you satisfied.
- If you crave sugar and other simple carbohydrates, fat is probably what your body needs.
- If you have trouble staying warm enough, fat will help regulate your body temperature.
- If your skin is dry, fat supports the glands that help keep skin and hair hydrated.

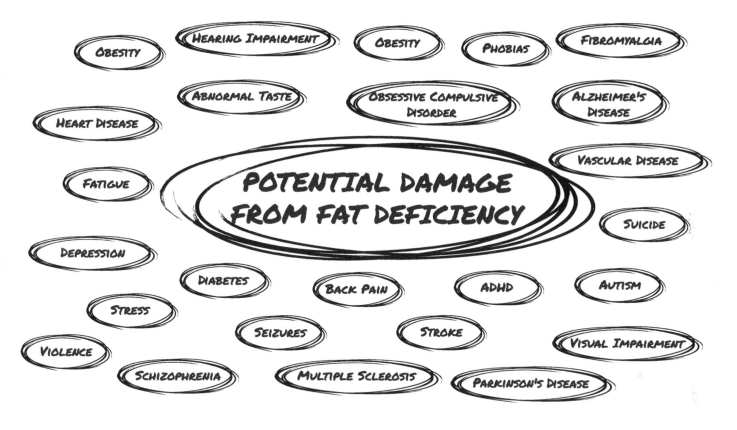

Fat should make up 50-60% of your daily calories.

- If you exercise faithfully, but still tire quickly, you may need to increase your fat to build stamina.

Three Kinds of Fats

We generally talk about three kinds of fats:

1. Polyunsaturated
2. Monounsaturated
3. Saturated

Bear in mind, however, that these are not distinct fats. Our sources of fat generally have *all* these fats in some proportion. That's why, in this section, we speak only about fats being high or low in one kind of fat, or having a high or low percentage of one of the fats.

Fat #1: Polyunsaturated Fats

Polyunsaturated fats occur naturally in nuts, seeds and fish. After processing, polyunsaturated fats are liquid, so many cooking oils like vegetable, canola and corn oil are primarily polyunsaturated.

Two polyunsaturated fatty acids have special significance for your brain: omega-3 fatty acids and omega-6 fatty acids.

1. Omega 3 Fatty Acids:

Our brains love omega-3 fatty acids, and so should you. These fatty acids:

- Decrease inflammation
- Improve neurological function
- Regulate moods and hormone production
- Reduce triglycerides, which are a type of fat in your blood
- Maintain good cell membranes—including cells in the brain
- Reduce the risk of an irregular heartbeat
- Slow the accumulation of plaque in your blood vessels, including those in your brain
- Help to lower your blood pressure

2. Omega-6 fatty acids

Omega-6 fatty acids are also essential to your health. In proper amounts, omega-6 fatty acids help control blood sugar, lower blood pressure and help in healing by contributing to the acute inflammatory response.

Ideally these fatty acids work together, but with a Standard American Diet (SAD), they are often at war.

Omega-6 fatty acids ⬆ **Inflammation**

Omega-3 fatty acids ⬇ **Inflammation**

Omega-6 and omega-3 fatty acids work together to start and stop inflammation

The battle between omega-6 vs. omega-3

Remember the SWAT analogy about inflammation? Omega-6, which causes inflammation, shows up like a SWAT team to deal with an emergency. Omega-3, which is anti-inflammatory, sends everyone home when the emergency has been dealt with.

Unfortunately, most of us get way too many omega-6 fatty acids in our diet in proportion to omega-3 fatty acids. When there's too much omega-6, the omega-3 can't get the crowd to go home when the emergency is over.

Our bodies need no more than two omega-6 fatty acids for every one omega-3 fatty acid. This preferred ratio of 2:1 allows the "shutting-down" process to work correctly. Anything higher—more omega-6 than you need—and the omega-3 can't do its essential work of shutting inflammation down.

How much more omega-6 do we get normally? In the Standard American Diet, we have a 20:1 ratio: *ten times more omega-6 than is good for us.*

No wonder we experience so much chronic inflammation!

Why is our ratio of omega-6 to omega-3 so bad?

First, we rely too heavily on vegetable oil in our diet. This includes canola, corn, soybean, and generic vegetable oil. Even olive oil has a 10:1 ratio of omega-6 to omega-3.

According to one report from the Pew Research Center published in 2010, Americans consume 36 pounds of vegetable oil every year—a quarter of our daily calorie intake and three times more than in the 1970s.[57] Soybean oil, used pervasively in restaurants, is currently the most significant source of omega-6 fatty acids in the United States.

Another reason for this imbalance is the practice of feeding domestic livestock cereal grains (such as corn) rather than grass. When we switched to raising cereal-fed livestock, we sacrificed the omega-3 fatty acids, leaving mostly omega-6 in our animal protein.

Because excessive omega-6 does so much damage to your health, getting more omega-3 into your diet is probably the single most important thing you can do to improve your source of fats.

How to Increase Your Intake of Omega-3

- Eat omega-3 rich fish at least once a week. Fish is your best dietary source of omega-3s. See the section on fish under protein for warnings about mercury in fish.

- Use most oils at room temperature.

- Olive oil is full of antioxidants and phytonutrients, and its omega-3 easily penetrates the cell membranes in your brain. This has a significant effect on brain clarity. If you cook at high heat with it, however, you may contribute to oxidation. It is best used at room temperature for dressing salads, drizzling on foods and dipping your bread.

- Eliminate your home use of corn oil, as well as sunflower, soybean or cottonseed oils. These are all high in omega-6s.

- Avoid processed or packaged foods, usually anything made with corn oil, soybean oil, and sunflower oils, or shortening, which are all high in omega-6 fatty acids.

- If you eat a lot of beef, lamb and other animal proteins, look for grass-fed options rather than grain-fed. Grain-fed livestock eat mostly soy- and corn-based diets, both of which contribute to high levels of omega-6 fatty acids in the meat. You can also purchase pork raised on animal feed that has

Page 69

been enriched with flax seed, making it higher in omega-3s.

- Choose a fish oil supplement that is high in omega-3. You probably get enough omega-6 in your diet already.

- Be careful in your choice of nuts. Most nuts have both omega-6 and omega-3. It's the ratio of each that matters. Among nuts, walnuts have one of the best ratios—4.2:1—while almonds have one of the worst—1500:1.

Fat #2: Monounsaturated Fatty Acids, or MUFAs

Monounsaturated fats have many health benefits. A diet high in MUFAs helps guard against heart disease. When you replace saturated fats with MUFAS, your blood pressure, blood cholesterol, triglycerides and your risk of cancer are likely to go down. Perhaps this is because MUFAs are so high in antioxidants and phytochemicals. Foods that are high in monounsaturated fats include olive oil, pumpkin seeds, avocados and nuts.

Fat #3: Saturated Fats

Typically, saturated fats are solid at room temperature. Highest concentrations are found in dairy products such as cheese, whole-fat milk and butter, and in meat protein such as beef, pork and others.

There's some controversy about whether saturated fats contribute to heart disease and other chronic inflammatory conditions like Alzheimer's dementia.

Olive Oil

Krill Oil
(Supplement)

Coconut Oil
(High in MCTs)

Culinary Algae Oil

Fish Oil
(High in Omega-3)

Oils that are good for you

For these reasons, I strongly suggest that you moderate the saturated fat in your diet, including dairy. Eat grass-fed, grass-finished beef in moderation.

Two foods high in saturated fats need special discussion.

Processed Meats

Processed meats are the worst source of saturated fats. They include hot dogs, bratwurst, pepperoni, salami, lunch meats—and yes, bacon.

The nitrosamines produced in most of these foods cause the liver to produce fats that are toxic to the brain. Your brain goes on full alert when it senses them, generating chronic inflammation. Studies associate these meats with a 42% higher risk of heart disease and a 19% higher risk of type 2 diabetes.[58]

For the sake of your brain, cut processed meat out of your diet. If you must indulge, eat only as a special treat.

This advice is not controversial. The World Health Organization, Mayo Clinic, the American Heart Association and most other health organizations agree that processed meats are harmful.

Coconut Oil: Good or Bad?

Check on the Internet, and you'll find incredible health claims for coconut oil. You'll also read warnings because it is mostly saturated fats.

So is it good for you or bad for you?

Coconut oil gets 87% of its calories from saturated fats (compared to 14% for olive oil and 63% for butter), and in most controlled trials, it increases bad cholesterol as much as other saturated fats.

Because of this, many reputable heart-related health organizations say to avoid it. At a minimum, I would advise using it sparingly. For the sake of your brain, you want to keep your heart happy. ***Happy heart, happy brain.***

At the same time, 13% of coconut oil has a special kind of fat called medium-chain triglycerides. These triglycerides offer many benefits:

- MCTs get used faster than other fats so are less likely to be stored by your body.
- MCTs break down into ketones, which your brain can use as fuel.
- MCTs cross the membrane of the mitochondria more quickly, giving you more energy.
- MCTs increase your good HDL cholesterol. Does this out-balance the rise in bad cholesterol that results from the saturated fat in coconut oil? Further research is necessary before we can answer that question.

Some people consider MCT so beneficial to the brain that they drink two tablespoons of coconut oil each morning, often mixed into their coffee. It's delicious.

When purchasing unprocessed coconut oil, look for organic, unrefined, virgin, cold-pressed coconut oil without added cottonseed and canola oils, sold in glass jars.

However, be careful. It's the MCTs, not the coconut oil, that helps your body, and the percentage of MCTs in coconut can vary dramatically—from as little as 13% to 100% in some designer coconut oils. If you can afford it, I recommend that you purchase 100% MCT oil derived from coconut oil. You'll get more of the benefits of medium-chain triglycerides and fewer of the problems associated with saturated fat.

Whatever You Do, Avoid All Added Trans Fats

The worst kind of fat for you is artificial trans fatty acids, commonly shortened to trans fats. They are so universally reviled that many restaurants, even fast-food restaurants, no longer use them, and after years of debate, the FDA recently removed trans fats from the Generally Recognized as Safe (GRAS) list. So artificial trans-fat usage has finally begun to decline.

It should be non-existent!

How trans fats came into being

Oil in its natural form (liquid at room temperature) breaks down rapidly, causing packaged foods to spoil easily—think rancid oil on popcorn, gluey biscuits, stale cookies. Stale foods didn't sell very well.

To solve this problem, in 1902 scientist Wilhelm Normann started adding hydrogen to vegetable oil so that packaged foods had a longer shelf life, and restaurants could use oil for deep frying without having to change it as often. Its use spread quickly.

The same oil that doesn't break down as easily on a shelf does not break down as readily in our bodies. It sits like an unwelcome invader, hindering our ability to make use of other proteins or fats and causing many other problems.

I hope the words "unwelcome invader" flipped the inflammation switch in your mind because, yes, our bodies go into full immune defense against trans fats, resulting in chronic inflammation and its many associated health problems. According to the Harvard T.H. Chan School of Public Health, for every 2% of calories you get from trans fats, your risk of heart disease increases by 23%.[59]

Trans fats and the brain

Trans fats increase inflammation in the brain, contributing to nerve cell destruction and cognitive decline. Trans fats also seem to disturb hormone production, inhibit production of omega-3 fatty acids which your brain needs to thrive, and reduce serotonin production, leading to depression, bad moods and aggressive behavior.

I strongly urge you to eliminate all manufactured trans fats from your diet.

How to avoid trans fats in your diet

For now, even when foods contain up to 0.5 gm of trans fats, companies can list the trans fats as 0 on the nutrition label. Even in small amounts, the damage from trans fats adds up quickly.

So always check the list of ingredients. The term *partially hydrogenated vegetable oil (PHVO)* is the giveaway. This ingredient = trans fats.

Here are some specific sources of trans fats (notice how many are processed foods):

- **Margarine and shortening:** Check the ingredients list for partially hydrogenated oils.
- **Store-bought baked goods, refrigerator dough, snacks, microwave popcorn, waffle and pancake mixes, crackers and cake mixes and frostings:** Most of these contain shortening, often made from PHVO. Some microwaved popcorn has 15 grams of trans fat per bag.

- **Frozen dinners and anything battered and fried in the frozen food aisle:** Trans fats give these foods a better "mouth feel," so producers continue to use at least a little. Brands that claim to be healthier do often avoid PHVOs entirely.

- **Pies and pie crusts:** PHVO helps to keep the crust flaky, so many manufacturers and restaurants continue to use it. Check labels at the grocery store, and ask at restaurants.

- **Restaurant/fast food breakfast sandwiches, and anything battered or fried:** If you must eat these salty, high-calorie foods, opt for chains that promise 0 trans fats (which legally only means less than 0.5 grams). If in doubt, ask what kind of oil they use. (And even with no trans fats, keep these foods as an indulgence.)

Summary Advice on Fats in Your Diet

- Increase omega-3 fatty acids.
- Avoid oils high in omega-6 fatty acids (vegetable, canola, corn oil).
- Oil is always healthier used at room temperature. Heating it produces harmful byproducts.
- You should store plant-based oils in a cool, dark place because light causes them to break down. Throw away any old, rancid, or spoiled oils.

- The best oil to cook with (if you must) is oil that is high in monounsaturated fat (omega-9 fatty acids). This oil is least affected by exposure to heat and oxygen.

- Moderate intake of foods high in saturated fat (from meat and dairy, mostly). Saturated fat contributes to a rise in cholesterol. It also lacks the protective qualities found in omega-3 fatty acids.

- Never eat trans fats—*ever*!

- If you use fresh, organic forms of these oils, your brain will thank you.

Protein, an Essential Nutrient

Protein is essential to every cell in your body. It helps build strong muscles and tissue, heals cells throughout your body and is a building block of skin and blood.

In the brain, protein is essential to the production of neurotransmitters. These chemicals carry signals from one brain cell to another and throughout the nervous system. Because of this, getting the right amount of protein increases mental clarity, memory and cognition; boosts your energy; helps regulate pain; reduces anxiety; initiates deep sleep; and makes you happier.

Since your brain needs a steady supply of protein, it's a good idea to space out your intake throughout the day. Doing so will help you feel full longer than carbohydrates do and may help you avoid the eating that leads to sugar spikes.

Too Much Protein

Most Americans get far more protein than necessary. Only about 20% - 25% of our calories each day needs to come from protein. That translates to 46 grams for women and 56 grams for men. However, if you are doing a lot of strength training (good for you!), you may need a little bit more protein, but be careful. Too much protein burdens your body.

Problems with Too Much Protein

These are especially true for meat-based protein:

- *Puts a strain on your kidneys:* Your kidneys have to process and eliminate the nitrogen byproducts that you get along with protein.

- *Causes problems in your GI tract:* All fiber comes from plant sources, and if you're overloading on animal-based proteins, you probably aren't getting the fiber you need. The resulting GI problems increase inflammation throughout your body.

- *Causes bad breath*

- *Causes weight gain*: Especially with high-fat animal-based protein

- *Accumulates LDL cholesterol in your blood:* This is the bad kind of cholesterol that increases your

risk of heart disease.

- *Can lead to many other illnesses*: These could include cancer, diabetes, heart disease and osteoporosis.

So as you think about the right kinds of protein, please remember that you also need the right *amount* of protein.

Good Sources of Protein

Fish

For your brain, adding seafood to your plant-based proteins is probably the best choice. Fish, especially fresh-caught salmon and sardines, have the omega-3 fatty acids your brain needs.

The following tips will help you with making the best seafood choices:

- Look for "Frozen-at-Sea" (FAS) for the freshest fish.
- Choose line-caught fish whenever possible.
- Fish raised in farms can be subject to contaminants. You can minimize these by removing the skin and trimming fat. Look for a label that says "low-density." This means the farmers raised them in uncrowded pens or tanks, with no antibiotics or hormones.
- Try to avoid fish higher on the food chain, like tuna, shark or swordfish, as they accumulate all the mercury and other toxins consumed by the smaller fish they eat.

- If you do buy tuna, avoid albacore, which is higher in mercury, and opt for skipjack tuna, used in most canned light tuna. Water-packed tuna retains more omega-3 fatty acids.
- Buy American. U.S. fisheries have been working ssshard to raise fish responsibly, but seafood from other countries can pose risks.

Plant-Based Protein

Some of the best plant-based proteins are beans and legumes. They give your body a good helping of fiber and are also very high in vitamins, minerals, fiber, antioxidants and many other healthy nutrients.[60]

If making beans and legumes at home, however, soak them thoroughly and cook them before eating. Proteins found in legumes and beans contain lectins, which are thought to damage the lining of your digestive system.

Nuts and seeds are nature's perfect snack food, as long as you don't eat too many! They provide protein, and several are good sources of omega-3. Some vegetables like spinach and broccoli also provide protein.[61]

Meat-based protein

Eat meat-based protein in moderation, including skinless cuts of chicken, turkey and duck; lean cuts of pork tenderloin; lean cuts of beef (for example, flank steak), lamb and buffalo. The fat in meat is saturated and could cause problems for your heart.

Try to purchase grass-fed and grass-finished meat

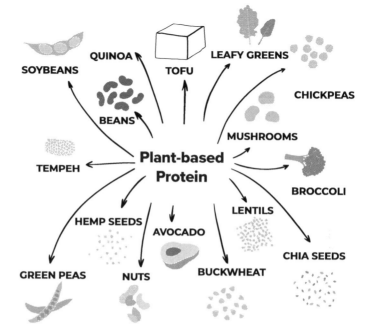

Make room in your diet for plant-based proteins.

(beef, lamb and buffalo) whenever possible. This "grass-finished" label indicates the stock has been fed grass throughout its life.

Typical feed used for livestock elevates omega-6 fatty acids. Grass-fed and finished livestock produce meat that contains more omega-3 fatty acids, which will help optimize brain function.

Bad Sources of Protein

Unfortunately, most Americans indulge in a diet that includes way too much of the wrong kinds of protein: highly marbled and fatty cuts of beef, pork and other meats, as well as cheese, creams and other high-fat dairy products.

Among the worst of these "bad" meats are the

processed ones like bacon, sausages, hot dogs and brats. These have a higher proportion of saturated fats, which can lead to cardiovascular diseases that damage your brain and have a high correlation with some kinds of cancer.

Avoid processed meats, whether salted, cured or smoked.

The Right Carbohydrates

Carbohydrates are essential to your health because they provide most of the energy your body needs to survive. That's why I began the chapter with a section on fruits and vegetables, which I call the "cornerstone of a good nutritional platform."

Even so, carbohydrates can cause serious problems for your brain if you choose the wrong ones. In Chapter 9, we emphasized (and reemphasized) the importance of avoiding added sugar. We will stress this again in the Chapter 14 and Chapter 18. Added sugar is the absolutely worst kind of carbohydrate you can choose to eat.

Here are three additional tips for choosing the right kinds of carbohydrates:

- *Choose whole carbohydrates:* Get most of your carbohydrates from the organic produce section of your grocery store or farmer's market. Whole grains, beans and legumes are also good for you.

- *Reject processed foods:* These are the carbohydrates found in baked goods, ice cream, French fries, sugary soft drinks, fruit juices, pastries and most desserts. You'll also need to be careful about foods you "process" at home such as mashed potatoes, casseroles with white pasta or white rice and of course anything made with added sugar. Make it a goal to fill your sugar bin less and less often.

- *Be careful with fruit that is high in sugar,* especially if you are monitoring your blood sugar. Check your blood sugar levels after eating these fruits, such as watermelon, grapes and pineapple, and avoid them if you must.

What about Gluten?

Gluten is a protein in wheat, rye or barley that acts as a glue to help foods hold their shape. You can find it in all the foods and drinks made with these grains, including most bread, beer, pasta and many other processed foods.

Of concern to your brain, gluten contributes to changes in the gut microbiome, and problems in your gut cause inflammation in your brain. This is especially true if you have any degree of gluten sensitivity or wheat allergy.

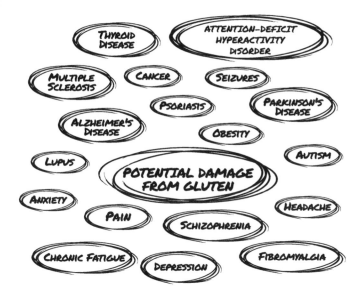

You may need to limit gluten

Why is Gluten Getting So Much Attention?

The gluten used in products today is not the same gluten encountered throughout most of history. Those who process foods have heavily engineered gluten through hybridization, and many of our bodies react to it with inflammation.

The pro-inflammatory responses that gluten causes contribute to many neurological, psychiatric and autoimmune diseases—and possibly even cancer.

How to Know if You Are Sensitive to Gluten

The test used to measure gluten sensitivity produces many false negatives. I therefore advise my patients to experiment on their own with a gluten-free diet. Many have experienced significant improvements in their overall health, especially in the areas included in the chart at left illustrating potential damage from gluten.

Be careful about starting a gluten-free diet, however. It can lead to lower levels of iron, calcium, fiber, folate, thiamin, riboflavin and niacin. Your doctor can advise you how to compensate for these if necessary.

Also, avoid processed gluten-free products as you would all processed foods.

How to Minimize Gluten in Your Diet

First, talk to your doctor. If you don't have celiac disease or an actual allergy, you may not want to eliminate foods that contain gluten completely. You can moderate them or, for the sake of your brain, consider them an indulgence. Here are some steps to do that:

1. **Limit or avoid wheat, barley and rye,** all of which contain gluten.

2. **Fill your diet with non-grain fruits and vegetables.** If you focus on these, you'll have less room for gluten-rich items.

3. **Choose alternative grains,** such as quinoa, millet, buckwheat, teff, gluten-free oats and amaranth.

Intermittent Fasting

Many religious traditions encourage fasting, and now scientific data agrees. Fasting can be beneficial for your emotional, spiritual and physical health.

I would like to acquaint you with intermittent fasting, but only as one option for your nutritional plan.

Intermittent fasting involves not eating for a certain number of hours each day or during certain days of the week. Some people fast for 12 hours, from dinner to breakfast. Some stretch this to 18 hours (dinner to lunch). Some fast only two days a week. Others fast every day.

Whatever you might choose, please talk to your doctor about *any* fasting, and especially intermittent fasting. Not everyone agrees with the benefits of intermittent fasting, especially for diabetics, and some people need to be on a strict eating program because of depression or other mental health issues.

Intermittent fasting may also cause rebound eating when the fast is over, elevate cortisol levels and increase food intolerances that cause inflammation.

That's why talking to your doctor is essential!

Benefits of Intermittent Fasting

Brain-Derived Neurotrophic Factor (BDNF)

Your brain has a category of proteins called **neurotrophins**. These help neurons survive, develop and function.

Remember BDNF from Chapter 6? Intermittent fasting and caloric restriction seem to elevate BDNF.[62] Its positive effect on BDNF is why intermittent fasting can be so valuable for your cognitive health—if your doctor approves.

Ketones and Their Effect on the Brain

The brain requires about 20% of the total energy your body uses, so a steady source is crucial. When fasting, the supply of glucose eventually stops, and your liver has to turn to a backup source. This source is the ketones found in fatty acids. This switch can help protect the brain.[63]

After a period of intermittent fasting, if you find that you are feeling calmer, more relaxed and energetic, it's probably the ketones. A ketogenic state makes your brain sharper and decreases the chance for stroke, multiple sclerosis, Parkinson's and even brain tumors.

Deliberately putting yourself into ketosis is a somewhat controversial decision, primarily because overworking your liver can lead to a condition called ketoacidosis. That's why I encourage you to talk to your doctor, who may have you moderate your intermittent fasting, especially if you have diabetes.[64]

Other Benefits of Intermittent Fasting

- *Lower levels of sugar in your blood:* After fasting, insulin more effectively communicates the need for your body to take up glucose from your blood.

- *Speeds up your metabolism:* Whatever you eat, your body will use more quickly.

- *Helps you lose weight:* Intermittent fasting encourages the body to burn up fat. During fasting, your body begins using fat for energy rather than sugars.

- *Decreases inflammation and primes your mitochondria:* Fasting also reduces oxidation, the damage that free radicals do in your body.

- *Spiritual benefits or self-enlightenment:* Many religious or philosophical systems encourage fasting so that when hunger strikes, people intentionally turn their thoughts to a higher power, to other people's needs or to their own need to cleanse the psyche of worries and toxic emotions. Used to this end, fasting can become a meaningful way to de-stress your life and achieve more peace within.

For more information about benefits of intermittent fasting, I encourage you to watch the 16-minute TED talk by Mark Mattson entitled "Why Fasting Bolsters Brain Power."

Choosing A System That Works for You

One of the simplest methods of intermittent fasting is to limit yourself to 600 calories a day, two days a week. You can eat your 600 calories at any time during the day or restrict your eating until the evening. On the other days, you can eat a normal diet of healthy foods.

I recommend 15 to 18 hours of fasting each day that you fast. If you stop eating at 6:00 p.m. and then wait to eat until 9:00 a.m. or 12:00 noon the next day, you would meet this standard.

Others choose to begin their fast after their noon meal, continuing through the night.

For information about this and other intermittent fasting plans, check out Kate Morin's Internet article on *The Daily Burn* entitled "5 Intermittent Fasting Methods: Which One is Right for You?"

Because the benefits of intermittent fasting take a while to kick in, once you've addressed the medical advice issue, it's crucial that you find a method you can sustain. Of course, you can always adjust your plan along the way.

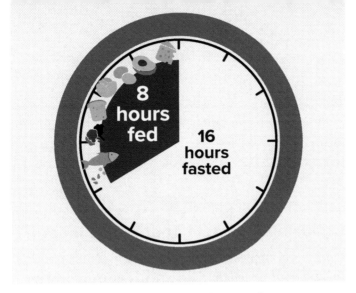

*16 hours of fasting to 8 hours of eating
is common in intermittent fasting*

When to Adjust Your Intermittent Fasting

Listen to your body so you can adjust your fasting plans as needed—or even abandon them entirely. Consider a change under the following circumstances:

- **When you can't stop eating during your off times:** Some people overindulge during their scheduled times for eating. The goal is healthier eating overall.

- **If the fasting disturbs your sleep:** You need to be able to fall asleep and stay asleep even when fasting. If this becomes difficult, adjust your fast. Lack of sleep alone will derail many efforts to improve your health.

- **If you are allowed 600 calories when you do intermittent fasting, but spend all these allotted calories on bad foods,** including processed and fast foods, added sugar, "diet" products and bad fats. Plan ahead so you can prepare healthier meals in advance.

Choose Health and Hope

Good food is medicine, and bad food is poison. You get to decide which kind you'll give your body and brain.

Good food mixes with oxygen and water in our mitochondria to make us energetic. Good food builds vigorous neurotransmitters, healthy immune systems, helpful enzymes and balanced hormones. Good food supports our longevity.

Bad food works against our health and accelerates our aging. By bad food I mean fast food, processed food, added sugar, stale and overused oils and too many fried foods. This is the Standard American Diet (SAD), and it will make you sick.

You can choose something better.

Spread the word. Healthy foods restore our health, reverse our fogginess and replace agitation with hope.

Chapter 11

Rid Your Body of Ultra Processed Foods

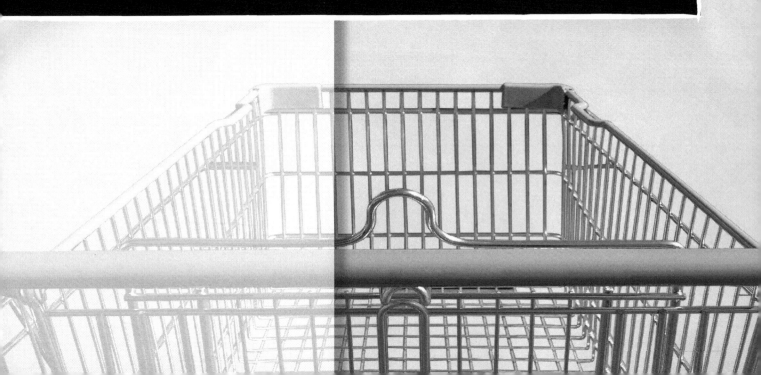

"Get people back into the kitchen and combat the trend toward processed food and fast food."

-Andrew Weil

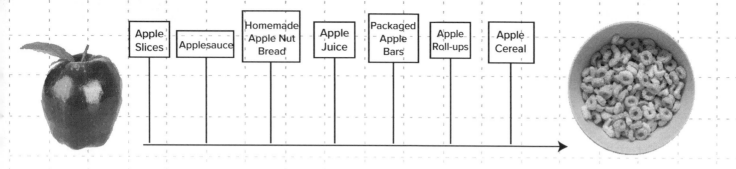

Almost every food item sold in your grocery store has been processed in some way. Someone has cleaned the fish, pasteurized the milk, trimmed or ground the meat and bagged many of the vegetables to look appealing on the shelf.

So when we speak of processed foods, we are actually talking about a spectrum from how the food would appear in nature to a minor item on an ingredient list.[65] From best to worst:

Fresh foods

You'll find these in the produce section. Apples, cucumbers, green beans as they appear in nature. All someone had to do was pick them and transport them to the store. For your health, always choose organic.

Minimally processed foods

These include bagged, cut or trimmed vegetables; shelled, unsalted nuts; and foods processed at their peak to lock in freshness and nutritional quality, such as canned tomatoes, frozen fruits and vegetables and canned tuna.

Foods cooked on location

A good bakery, a deli that produces fresh salads and serves them with fresh salad dressings, a sandwich shop that uses fresh, homemade ingredients—these approximate the "processing" you can do at home to produce healthy meals. Be careful to check, however, that their standards are as high as yours, including their use of fresh, organic oils.

Ultra-processed foods

These include ready-made foods produced at a factory, such as salad dressings, yogurt with fruit, jarred pasta sauce and packaged cookie dough and frozen cakes. Snack items like crackers and chips fit this category, as do most deli meats. The most heavily processed foods include frozen pizza, microwaveable dinners and factory-packaged desserts and cookies.

These foods have been made for you by a company, following a recipe that often includes added salt, refined sugar, fat that can sit for a long time on the shelf and unhealthy additives. Unfortunately, researchers estimate that Americans get up to 60% of their calories from these ultra-processed foods.[66]

Judiciously using processed food—even ultra-processed food—can contribute to less stress in your life (which is good). But the more you can remove them from your life, the better. Remember you can use simple recipes and techniques to cook at home and still keep things convenient.

A Word of Caution When Reading Food Ingredients

Health-food enthusiasts are fond of saying that if you can't recognize what an ingredient is, it must be bad for you. Turn a wary eye on this advice. You may not recognize cyanocobalamin or Streptococcus thermophiles. The first is Vitamin B12 and the second is a probiotic that can have many health benefits.

If there's an ingredient on the food label you don't recognize, do yourself a favor and look it up on your smartphone to find out what it is.

Ultimately, unrecognizable ingredients are *not* the reason processed foods are unhealthy.

The *Real* Reasons Why Ultra-Processed Food Can Be Bad for Your Health

- *Too much sugar*: Studies estimate that Americans get 500 calories a day from refined sugars—most of it sneaking in through processed foods. (See Chapter 9.) Too much sugar will damage your brain cells.

- *Bad fats*: Processed foods are a big reason why we get way too much omega-6 in our diet. Omega-6 fats increase inflammation and battle against omega-3 fats which our brains need. Also, some manufacturers still use trans fats, which are extremely bad for you. (See Chapter 10.)

- *Way too much salt*: If you are trying to be healthy, you would never add the amount of salt that food manufacturers do. They use it to make food more appealing, increase shelf life and add texture.

- *Fewer phytochemicals*: Processing destroys these important chemical compounds in fruits, vegetables and other plant-based foods. Phytochemicals protect your body from disease, toxins and other dangers.

- *Limit enzyme efficiency*, which causes problems for your brain and your gut. (See Chapter 18.)

- *Too easy*: Would you eat potato chips as often if you had to make them yourself? What about ice cream or donuts? A friend of mine, who grew up overseas, told me that in her home, donuts were a once-a-year event because they took so much time and effort to make. Now she can grab a few every time she pulls into a gas station.

- *Designed to entice you*: Food manufacturers are under no obligation to keep you healthy. Because most of all they want to make a sale, they create products with too much sugar, salt and the wrong kinds of fats.

- *Fewer nutrients*: Often the processing destroys the natural vitamins and minerals that are in whole foods. To make up for this, manufacturers add synthetic nutrients, but they are a poor substitute.

- **Less fiber**: Processing often strips fiber from food. This leaves you satisfied for a shorter time. (Ever heard of "hangry"?) Again, manufacturers are happy when you buy more.

Additives

For some people, *additives* is a bad word and should be avoided at all costs. However, people have been using additives in their food for millennia. Yogurt, pickles, fermented foods like sauerkraut and kimchi (which are good for your gut) and wine all depend on additives.

Some additives have even saved lives, according to Robert Gravani, Ph.D. food chemist from Cornell University. *Raise your hand*, he says, *if you know someone with pellagra? We eradicated this disease by adding niacin to bread products and flours. How about goiters? We wiped out this disease by adding iodine to our salt.*[67] So not all additives are bad.

In today's world, however, it pays to be careful about additives. Food has become over-populated with additives, mostly to increase shelf life, enhance taste and appearance or cut production costs.

The FDA monitors food additives, but the best they can say about any additive is that it is "Generally Regarded as Safe." In my mind, this is not the most convincing endorsement!

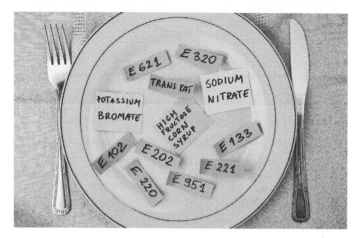

Additives that don't belong on your plate

Some common additives, such as food dyes, sodium benzoate, MSG and potassium sorbate, may cause allergic reactions (in other words, immune responses). Other additives, such as carrageenan, generate a lot of discussion as to their value with no resolution in sight.

But some additives are genuinely harmful to you:

- **Nitrates and nitrites**: These additives become a problem when added to processed meats. In the presence of protein and exposed to high heat (like frying, or grilling), they can end up as nitrosamines, a known carcinogen. (Nitrosamines are the primary carcinogen in tobacco smoke.)[68] In time, nitrosamines can contribute to Alzheimer's and cognitive decline. A 2009 study at Rhode Island Hospital found a "substantial link" between food with increased levels of nitrates and deaths from diseases like Alzheimer's, Parkinson's and type 2 diabetes.[69]

- **Trans fats, also known as partially hydrogenated vegetable oil**: This is an additive used in margarine, pastries, frozen foods, cookies, nondairy creamers, fast food and many more items. Even the FDA considers this unsafe and has instituted a plan for removing it from the market.

- *Yellow #5 and #6 Food Dyes*: Though still controversial, several studies link these dyes to learning problems in children. In response, Norway and Sweden have banned the dyes, and other countries in Europe require a warning on the food label.
- *BHA*: This is one of the additives used to keep food from spoiling. The U.S. Department of Health and Human Services classifies BHA as "reasonably anticipated to be a human carcinogen."[70] I recommend avoiding both BHA and BHT.

When you avoid processed foods, you are more than likely also avoiding food and drink that is full of harmful additives like nitrates and nitrites, preservatives, artificial coloring and flavoring. This will help you avoid fatty liver disease, diabetes, heart disease, cancer and cognitive impairment.

Making this change is straightforward and yet challenging. You can do it! Your brain will thank you.

How to Cut Down on Processed Foods

- *Do your own "processing"*: Cook at home, using ingredients you know and trust.
- *Add fresh foods to your meals.*
- *Stop eating processed meats*: Look for deli meats that are free of additives and preservatives and nitrate- and nitrite-free bacon and other meats.
- *Cook extra to create your own frozen meals*: Yours can have better ingredients than a factory's.
- *Avoid pre-packaged baked goods*: Instead, buy freshly made baked goods at a bakery where someone has used real ingredients without preservatives.
- *Cut out fast food* whenever possible, and always avoid fried options and processed meats.
- *Cut out frozen prepared foods* such as frozen dinners, frozen pies and frozen hash browns.
- *Buy food with no more than five ingredients*: A good rule of thumb, but not a fixed rule. There will always be exceptions.
- *Be careful where you eat out*: Choose restaurants that offer healthier menu selections.
- *Purchase 100% organic items*: When labeled "organic," foods cannot contain artificial preservatives, colors and flavors. Just be careful to wash your organic fruits and vegetables, an essential step in food safety.

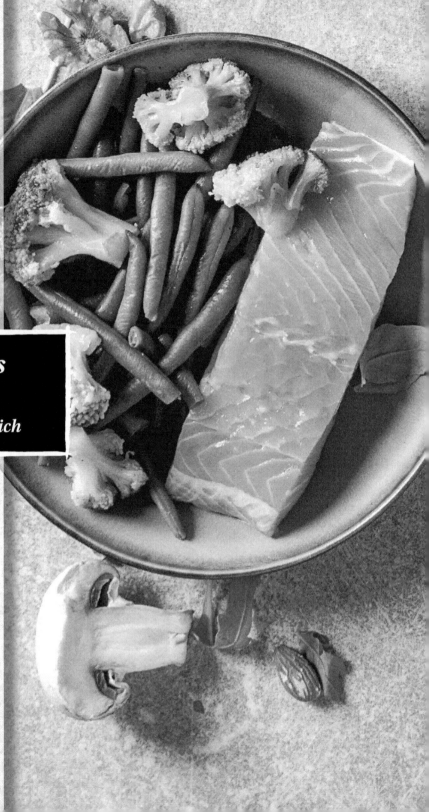

Chapter 12

Rid Your Body of Nutritional Gaps

> *"A healthy outside starts from the inside."*
>
> - Robert Urich

I have already said, but I want to stress it again: If you are considering the use of supplement, check with your doctor before you add them to your diet.

Some of the supplements (selenium, for example) can cause problems when taken in excess. Others have side effects that can be harmful (such as too much magnesium if you have kidney disease).

The Importance of Vitamins, Minerals and Cofactors

Vitamins help your body stay energetic, healthy and resistant to disease and infection. Minerals also help your body function properly. Cofactors and coenzymes work with your body's enzymes to complete reactions throughout your body. The chart on the following page explains how these nutrients contribute to your health.

It is always better to get these essential nutrients through your diet because they are more balanced and biologically active when you get them from food rather than from pills.

Many of the vitamins, minerals and cofactors that I discuss here, however, are at very minimal levels in the American diet. At least for a short period, until your overall diet improves, one or more of the following supplements may be beneficial.

Please, discuss the use of supplements with your primary care physician before you start taking them.

The following table describes supplements, their national sources, plus health benefits and notes.

TABLE: Supplement – Its Natural Source, and Health Effect

Supplement	Natural Source	Health Benefit/Notes
Acetyl-L-carnitine	• Beef, lamb, chicken, fish and dairy products—red meat is better • Supplements	• Helps the body produce energy • Crosses the blood-brain barrier to reduce oxidative stress and remove toxins • Helps produce neurotransmitters in the brain • Keeps blood flow in the brain healthy • Some evidence of improved memory in the elderly
Alpha Lipoic Acid	• Present in low levels in food like spinach, broccoli, yams, potatoes, yeast, tomatoes, Brussels sprouts, carrots, beets and rice bran • Red meat • Supplements	• Strong antioxidant • Fights cell decay • Helps turn food into energy • Can reach all parts of the cell because it is both fat and water soluble • Called the "universal antioxidant"
Vitamin B1 (Thiamine)	• Nuts • Green peas • Navy, black and pinto beans • Edamame • Sunflower, chia, pumpkin and squash seeds • Asparagus • Fortified bread • Fish and lean pork • Supplements	• Helps with energy production • Maintains cardiovascular function • Helps eye health and prevention of cataracts • Improves brain function • Helps maintain the integrity of the myelin sheaths

Supplement	Natural Source	Health Benefit/Notes
Vitamin B2 (Riboflavin)	• Beef liver • Lamb • Milk • Yogurt • Mushrooms • Spinach • Nuts • Multivitamins	• Serves as a coenzyme, helping enzymes do their work • Helps cells use energy
Vitamin B6 (pyridoxine)	• Bananas • Carrots • Spinach • Peas • Potatoes • Fish • Poultry	• Helps keep your skin healthy • Detoxifies the liver • Improves cognitive function • Supports eye health • Helps improve anemia • Helps maintain a healthy metabolism
Vitamin B9 (folic acid or folate)	• Green leafy vegetables • Fruit • Eggs • Legumes	• Helps prevent congenital disabilities • Helps prevent premature aging • Helps prevent heart attacks • May help combat depression • Supports red blood cell production

Supplement	Natural Source	Health Benefit/Notes
Vitamin B12 (cobalamin or cyanocobalamin)	• Animal sources: fish, meat, poultry, eggs, dairy products • Fortified cereals	• Supports myelin, the fatty substance that surrounds nerve cells • Helps make DNA • Helps keep red blood cells healthy • B12 is not available from plant-based foods, so people following a vegan diet must use supplements.
CO-Q10 (Coenzyme Q10)	• Supplements • Organ meat • Meat • Nuts	• Cofactor that helps enzymes do their work • Present in all mitochondria, helping to produce ATP • Powerful antioxidant • Production in your body decreases with age
Glutathione	• You make glutathione in your body, but you can support production by eating sulfur-rich foods like garlic, onions, broccoli, kale, spinach, cabbage, cauliflower • Supplements	• Powerful antioxidant • Helps to control inflammation • Counteracts stress • Limits neurodegeneration

Supplement	Natural Source	Health Benefit/Notes
Magnesium	• Dark leafy vegetables • Nuts and seeds • Beans and lentils • Whole grains • Avocados	• Helps activate nerve channels that keep brain synapses supple • Avoid alcohol, soft drinks and the wrong kind of fats which can block your body's ability to absorb magnesium. • Some evidence for magnesium L-threonate as the supplement of choice • Always discuss supplements with your doctor
Manganese	• Leafy vegetables • Grains • Nuts • Teas	• Too much manganese can be harmful to your health • Part of the principal antioxidant enzyme in the mitochondria • Usually part of a multivitamin
N-Acetyl Cysteine (NAC)	• Sulfur-rich food • Supplement	• Your body converts NAC to cysteine which is a precursor to glutathione. The health properties of glutathione are listed above.
Selenium	• Eggs • Mushrooms • Nuts • Meats, poultry and fish • Whole grains	• Powerful antioxidant • Promotes immune system health • Supports optimal thyroid function • Be careful not to get too much selenium. The recommended range is 55 to 400 micrograms per day.

Supplement	Natural Source	Health Benefit/Notes
Taurine	• Fish • Meat • Shellfish • Dairy • Poultry	• Improves memory by increasing the survival of neurons in the hippocampus • Levels decrease with age, but you can increase them with supplements • Improves cardiac function
Vitamin C	• Fruits, especially citrus • Vegetables	• Powerful antioxidant • Helps the healing process • Necessary for the formation of blood vessels, cartilage, muscle and collagen in bones • Helps the body absorb and store iron • Helps guard against cancer, cardiovascular disease and macular degeneration
Vitamin D	• Salmon • Tuna • Fortified dairy products • Beef liver • Egg yolks	• Necessary for the body to absorb calcium • Helps prevent cancer • Reduces risk of multiple sclerosis, osteoporosis, psoriasis and dementia

Supplement	Natural Source	Health Benefit/Notes
Vitamin E	• Almonds • Raw seeds • Spinach • Kale • Mustard and turnip greens	• A strong antioxidant • Protects membranes from oxidation • May prevent the loss of DHA, an essential omega-3 fatty acid in the brain
Zinc	• Whole grains • Dairy products • Fortified cereals • Seafood • Lean meats • Poultry • Legumes • Nuts and seeds	• Boosts the immune system • Improves wound healing • Prevents infections

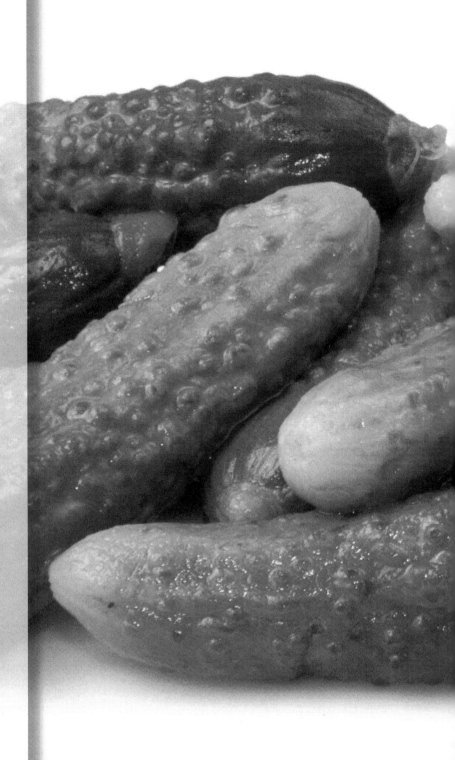

Chapter 13

Rid Your Body of Excess Salt

*Too much salt,
a pickled brain?*

You have probably heard that too much salt increases your risk of heart disease and strokes.

Did you know too much salt can also increase your risk of Alzheimer's? This evidence-based concern is one more reason to limit your salt.[71]

Your Body Treats Excess Salt as a Threat

Scientists studying the effects of a high-salt diet in mice discovered something interesting. The high-salt diet raised the levels of an inflammatory mediator called IL-17 inside the mice's small intestines. The increased levels of IL-17 was an adaptive immune response, which means the inflammatory response stayed in the intestines as long as the high-salt diet continued.[72]

As always, this severe and chronic inflammation affected other nearby cells. One result was that less nitric oxide was produced in the cells lining the mice's blood vessels.

Nitric oxide keeps the linings of the blood vessels relaxed, so the high-salt diet ultimately resulted in hardened arteries. These stiffened arteries inhibited the transport of blood throughout the mice. This meant the cells received less oxygen.

That included cells in the brain.

In mice on a high-salt diet, blood flow decreased as much as 25% to the hippocampus and 28% to the cortex. The hippocampus, remember, is the memory center of the brain. The ability of these mice to recognize objects, run through a maze and build nests decreased dramatically. Their brains just couldn't function well with all that salt.

Animal studies don't always translate perfectly to humans. Even so, it seems likely that too much salt in your diet could begin choking off blood to your brain as well.

This spells danger because blood is how your brain gets nutrients and energy. A three-year study by researchers in Canada supported this, showing a correlation between older adults on a low-salt diet and better cognitive performance.[73] Research also supports the claim that decreasing salt intake will improve your cognitive function. [74]

More research is needed, but according to available studies, you should add cognitive health to the list of reasons why limiting salt intake is better for your health.

How to Limit Salt in Your Diet

1. *Prepare your own food.* Most of the salt in the American diet comes from processed foods, which include restaurant/fast foods, snacks, mixes, baked goods and more—basically, anything prepared or partially prepared by someone else. So purchase fresh, unprocessed foods, including fruits, vegetables and meat that you can prepare yourself.

2. *Modify the amount of salt you add both when cooking and at the table.* Salt is an acquired taste, and you can unlearn it. Decrease it slowly, but be persistent. Experts say it could take six to eight weeks, but eventually, you will enjoy food with less salt.

You will also need to be on the lookout for unexpected sources of salt:

-   *Read labels* if you must purchase processed foods to find the lowest salt options. Condiments, salad dressings and other sauces are often high in sodium.
-   *Rinse canned foods* to remove as much salt as possible.
-   *At fast-food restaurants* (if you must eat there), train your mind to think, *Danger, danger, danger.*
-   *For those indulgent moments* (pizza!), enjoy yourself, but eat less than you usually would. That way you can at least limit the salt you're eating before you get back on track!

Chapter 14

Rid Your Body of Harmful Drinks

"Water is the driving force in nature."

-Leonardo DaVinci

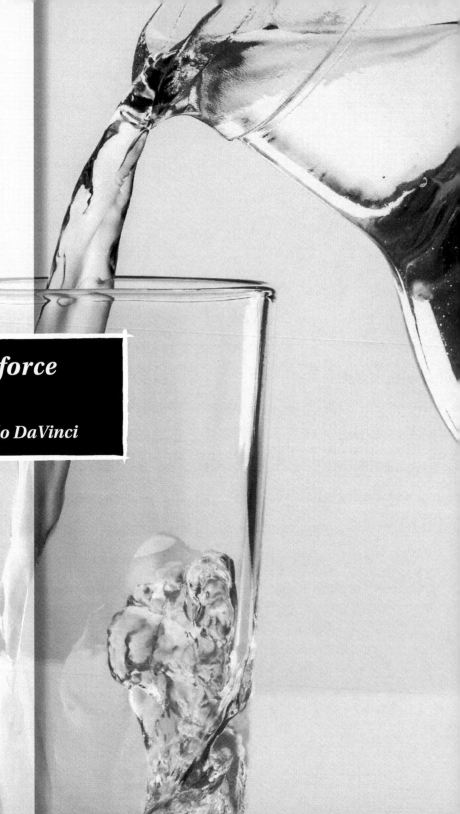

Water, The Best Drink of All

Adequate hydration is essential for human health and well-being, and clean water is one of the best ways to hydrate.

Water provides an environment in your body for millions of essential biological reactions. Water allows your body to maintain blood volume, regulate temperature and transport necessary materials throughout the body—including to and throughout your brain.

Water is also the highway that allows your body to remove toxins you have picked up from the environment or produced inside your body.

What is "Adequate" Hydration?

Your brain needs water, and if you don't get enough, your brain lets you know with a mild to moderate headache.

The headache occurs because a dehydrated brain temporarily retracts from the skull to conserve function, and this hurts. (You can quickly fix this headache by drinking water.)

So how much do you need to avoid dehydration?

The Internet has a lot of answers to this question—8 cups a day, 10 cups a day or even more. But experts warn that we are all unique, and our intake of fluids is too complex to set a firm standard.

If you live in a hot climate, exercise often, eat a salty snack, have an infection or are just getting older, you might need more.

You also may need less depending on where you live and what you eat and drink. Soup, green tea, juicy fruits, milk, lettuce and tomato sauces all have a lot of water, and add to your daily hydration.

In our rush to get enough fluids each day, we forget that drinking too much water can lead to dangerously low levels of sodium. This condition is called hyponatremia and it can lead to brain damage and death.

Then how much should I drink?

Instead of a certain amount of water each day, most experts now advise "drinking your thirst."[75] In other words, when you feel thirsty, drink water.

You can generally tell from your urine if you are getting enough fluids. If your urine is light yellow or almost clear, you're doing well. If it gets darker you are probably dehydrated and need to drink.

Hazards in the Water

When it comes to Alzheimer's, however, the quality of water you drink is probably more important than the amount of water. Sadly, water today is often not as pure as it should be.

As previously stated, the blood-brain barrier is a covering around the blood vessels in your brain. This barrier protects the brain by filtering out unwanted intruders.

Blood is mostly water (92%). If you drink water containing harmful substances, they will likely end up in your blood.

When this water reaches the brain's blood vessels, the contaminants can overwhelm the blood-brain barrier so that it fails to keep contaminants out of the brain. Once past the barrier, these contaminants damage neurons, create inflammation and generally throw the brain into turmoil.

That's why the quality of the water you drink is so vital to maintaining proper brain function.

Groundwater Contamination

More than half of U.S. residents get their water from wells and springs, including many people with public water systems in cities and towns. Unfortunately, groundwater is frequently contaminated.

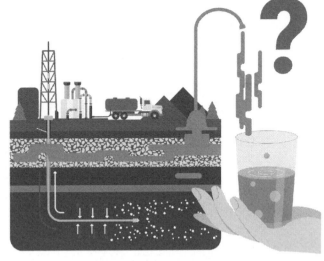

Groundwater can pick up a lot of contaminants on its way to your glass.

- Rain, snow and fog, the source of most groundwater, pick up contaminants from the air.
- This same precipitation picks up more contaminants as it seeps into the ground. These include agricultural pesticides and fertilizers, roadway oil and salts and industrial waste.
- Sometimes our groundwater becomes contaminated by the runoff and leaching from public landfills, regardless of how carefully these are monitored.
- Once underground, further contamination from leaky tanks of propane and gasoline or from sewage can seep into our groundwater.

In cities and towns, water treatment plants work hard to remove these contaminants. If you get your water directly from a well or natural spring, installing a residential water filtration system will help with these contaminants.

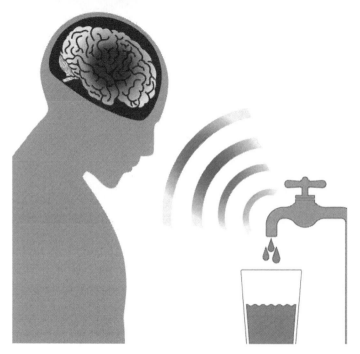

What's in your water could cause inflammation in your brain.

You can remove additional contaminants by using a water filtration pitcher for tap water or another personal water filtration system in your home. It's best to have a mixture of both ion exchange and activated carbon technology.

The Problem with Chlorine

In some countries, a glass of water can make people deathly ill because the water contains microbes that cause diseases like cholera, dysentery and typhoid. In America, we usually remove these microbes by adding chlorine, a highly effective disinfectant, to the water.

If used judiciously, chlorine saves lives, but today chlorine's reach goes much further than just water. We use it in household cleaners, in swimming pools, in the food industry as a cleaner, in bleached coffee filters and paper towels. It seems to be everywhere.

Too much chlorine can affect your whole body, from your heart to your skin, hair, liver, lungs, and *also your brain*. It contributes to low sperm count, miscarriages and congenital malformations. There's also a strong correlation between too much chlorine and kidney problems and bladder and colon cancer.[79]

What you can do: A water filtration pitcher or dispenser can remove much of the chlorine that remains after water treatment, either at your well or at your public water treatment plant. Please be sure to change the filter as recommended.

The Dilemma of Fluoride

Fluoride has been called "nature's cavity fighter." It strengthens enamel as teeth develop, and it helps fight tooth decay. The return on investment is excellent—up to $38 for every $1 invested. For the sake of dental health, many health authorities consider fluoridation beneficial at the low levels used in communities.[76]

I want to be fair and transparent, so I acknowledge this benefit right up front. However, given its other effects on your body and especially your brain, I seriously question whether fluoride in our water is worth it.

- Fluoride is one of the EPA's top 100 chemicals that may contribute toxic effects on the brain's development.
- It accumulates in the brain and, based on animal studies, is linked to a decrease in learning.
- Fluoride has also been shown to contribute to an increase in aluminum in the brain and the formation of beta-amyloid deposits.[77]

It seems clear that avoiding fluoride will decrease your risk of Alzheimer's. Why take the chance?

I suggest you at least purchase one of the following: a water filtration pitcher, a system that removes fluoride or spring water to drink.

And if you are concerned about your dental health, cutting added sugar out of your diet will greatly improve that and your cognitive future!

Why not to drink bottled water

Bottled water has grown into a $60 billion industry worldwide, with spring water and purified tap water leading in sales worldwide. People enjoy the convenience, taste and accessibility of bottled water, and in emergencies, bottled water can be a lifesaver. As a rule, however, you may want to avoid bottled water.

First, there are the environmental problems caused by plastic bottles. Making the bottles uses 17 million barrels of oil annually.[78] The average American uses 167 disposable water bottles each year but recycles only 38.[79]

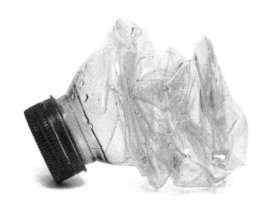

Plastic bottles create both environmental and health problems.

Fortunately, many companies are working diligently to come up with plastic bottles that can be sustainably produced and are biodegradable—but the greater hazard to your cognitive health comes from the BPA in plastic bottles.

BPA: Many plastic bottle manufacturers use BPA (bisphenol A) to make bottles more robust. It is also used to in can linings, in plastic wraps and cash register receipts.

BPA is a known estrogen disruptor. This means they interfere with the finely choreographed dance of hormones in your body.

After leaching into the water in bottles,[80] BPA gets absorbed by our bodies where it mimics estrogen. Not only does it cause "reproductive toxicity" (wow), it also disrupts our cognitive health. I explain endocrine disruptors in more depth in Chapter 21.

You may not have noticed this problem. That's because it builds over time—it's sneaky.

"BPA-free" labels: In response to criticism and

concerns, many manufacturers have switched to bisphenol S (BPS) or bisphenol F (BPF) to make their plastic. This allows them to slap a "BPA-free" label on their products.

Don't be fooled! These alternative softeners are just as bad for your hormones.[81]

What you can do:

- Use glass or stainless steel tumblers for drinking.
- Never microwave in plastic because heat encourages the chemicals to break down and leach into your food. Instead, use glass, ceramic or porcelain in a microwave oven.
- For the same reasons, avoid drinking from a water bottle that has been sitting in a hot car. The heat can turn the water into a BPA soup.
- Avoid canned foods. Many food companies use cans lined with BPA-containing resin.
- Though less dangerous than heating in plastic, you may also want to avoid freezing foods in plastic.

Bottom line:

Carry a refillable glass or stainless steel bottle. You can even purchase a personal water filtration device to use with your stainless steel or glass bottle. You'll be protecting yourself, the environment and your wallet!

One Last Problem Related to Water

It isn't only the water we drink that allows chemicals to enter our bodies. When we bathe or shower in hot water, the heat opens the skin's pores. This allows contaminants like chlorine and chloramines to enter our bodies through the skin.

Water in the bath or shower also mists and vaporizes from the heat, allowing you to inhale the contaminants. As you enjoy your hot bath, you could be absorbing many more contaminants than drinking unfiltered tap water.[82]

What you can do:

- If possible, purchase a whole-house water filtration system.
- For your showers, you might purchase a shower head filtration system, preferably one that uses Vitamin C to neutralize the chlorine and chloramines.
- For your bath, you can purchase Vitamin C tablets that will remove the chlorine.

Besides Water, Good Things to Drink for Your Health

- *Green tea* is high in antioxidants. In one study, two cups of green tea a day lowered evidence of cognitive decline by 50% (not conclusive, but insightful).[83]

- **Turmeric tea** is high in antioxidants and helps defend against metabolic disease. Mix ½ to 1 teaspoon turmeric powder in a cup of warmed almond milk (with a little honey if necessary). Finish with a pinch of black pepper, which is essential for absorption.
- **Smoothies** made with mostly kale, spinach, broccoli and berries are high in antioxidants. Add some ground flax seeds and chia seeds for good measure. Just be careful of smoothies that are mostly fruit. They have a high sugar content.

Drinks that Can Harm You

Caffeine

Caffeine is the number one neuroactive drug on the planet. In the US, we ingest around 12 million pounds of caffeine each year just through coffee.

The good news:

Some studies suggest that caffeine, which increases alertness and concentration, can actually lower your risk of Alzheimer's because it is such a potent antioxidant.

Researchers at Indiana University have also been investigating the ability of caffeine to combat the beta-amyloid plaques that can accumulate in the brain.[84] Others suggest that caffeine can block receptors that contribute to tau tangles.[85]

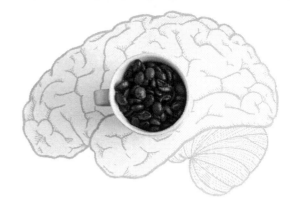

Caffeine can both help and harm your brain

The bad news:

Caffeine can also cause insomnia, and good sleep is much more important to your health than any benefits provided by caffeine. In addition, caffeine-induced anxiety contributes to stress, which makes it harder to guard against inflammation. Caffeine can also contribute to restlessness, tremors and fear, as well as elevated or irregular heartbeats.

Additionally, coffee that has not been stored carefully can develop toxic chemicals caused by mold. Decaf coffee tends to have higher levels, and in general, coffee that tastes bitter probably has mold.

So is caffeine good or bad for you?

It all depends on how you react to caffeine. Some people metabolize caffeine quickly. They drink coffee late at night and still drop off to sleep easily. For them, the benefits of caffeine probably outweigh the negatives.

Others metabolize coffee slowly. (*"No coffee for me after 3:00 p.m. or I'll never get to sleep tonight."*) For them the negatives may be worse than the benefits.

Bottom line:

Pay attention to your body's response to caffeine, and adjust your intake accordingly. If you do drink coffee, choose a high-quality, caffeinated coffee and store it in a clean, dry place. Discard coffee that tastes bitter.

Fruit Juice

An update for those of us who grew up in the 50s, 60s and 70s: Fruit juice is not healthy. Fruit juices do have some vitamins and nutrients, but in the eyes of many nutritionists, any benefit is overshadowed by the looming monster of sugar in fruit juices.

The problems with fruit juice

- *No fiber:* The fiber is in the pulp, but after processing, juice loses that advantage. One natural orange has about 3 grams of fiber. Most fruit drinks don't have any pulp at all. Even orange juice with pulp has negligible dietary fiber.

- *No fruit skin:* The skin is a vital source of nutrients in fruit. The skin often includes essential carotenoids and flavonoids.

- *Too much sugar:* Any good that remains after processing doesn't make up for the fruit juices' concentration of sugar. Put a glass of apple juice and the same sized-glass of soda next to it. The juice has 39 grams of sugar and the soda 40 grams. Soda—bad. Fruit juice—just as bad.

- *Too easy:* Eating fruit requires chewing, which slows down your eating and allows your body to start digesting the food. Juice goes down very quickly, so it's easy for your body to move the sugar into your bloodstream—sugar spike!

- *The quantity:* At one time, people had a small glass of orange juice in the morning for the Vitamin C. Now, we drink fruit juice as an alternative to water—a large tumblerful to slake our thirst. So not just a sugar spike, a *big* sugar spike.

- *The calories:* Sugary drinks, including fruit juices, are among the most fattening foods in existence.[86] Ironically, even though they are full of calories, they do not satisfy our hunger.

- *Loss of nutrients:* During processing, the juice loses nutrients, so much so that manufacturers often add vitamins back into the juice after processing. The juice also loses nutrients during storage.

- *Inflammation:* Remember that the amount of sugar in the fruit juice, especially in the absence of fiber, can increase inflammation.

- *Brain shrinkage:*[87] In the end, drinking your sugar can result in smaller brain volume and poorer memory function. Train yourself to hear alarm bells whenever you reach for *any* sweet drink.

Instead of juice, choose real fruit!

Sugared and Diet Drinks

Sugared drinks, including soft drinks, sports drinks and any of the other formulations manufacturers create, have way too much sugar and are highly addictive.

The evidence that sugary drinks promote weight gain and all its associated health problems is pretty conclusive.[88] Easily digested, sugared drinks contribute to insulin resistance and heart problems, increased risk of cancer and dental issues. They cause so many health problems that some people are pushing for a tax on sugared drinks similar to the tax on alcohol.

My advice—***Run from these sugary drinks!*** Your brain (and your body) will thank you.

Diet drinks have a close association with obesity and other metabolic problems like diabetes, as well as cardiovascular diseases and stroke. Scientists suggest these correlations are due to the damage soft drinks do in the gut and the desire for real sugar that seems to follow the use of artificial sweeteners.[89]

If you do indulge in soft drinks, please do so rarely, and resist the sugar cravings that will probably follow.

Alcohol

If you have ever drunk a little too much alcohol, you have probably experienced some of the effects alcohol has on the brain: difficulty walking, slurred speech, slower reaction times, blurred vision and impaired memory.

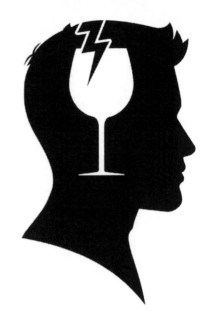

For your brain, drink alcohol only in moderation.

It's probably not a surprise, then, to learn that alcohol consumption could increase your risk for developing Alzheimer's later in life.

According to a 2013 study, 78% of people diagnosed with some disorder related to alcohol also displayed a form of Alzheimer's or brain-related disease (as well as many other serious problems!).[90]

In another study, researchers discovered a link between drinking six or more glasses of alcohol per day and a threefold increase in Alzheimer's risk.[91]

For those who already have Alzheimer's, consuming alcohol can hasten their decline.[92]

In fairness, alcohol consumption often accompanies other risk factors like smoking. Even so, experts are confident that alcohol has a significant role in this increased risk.

How Alcohol Affects the Brain

- Alcohol produces acetaldehyde, which is toxic to brain cells.
- It raises blood pressure, which is very bad for your brain.
- Alcohol alters the genes of microglial cells that help to clean out beta-amyloid after it does its protective work.[93] (See Chapter 5.)
- Consuming too much alcohol prevents neurons from regenerating. When neurons can't regenerate, the brain shrinks in size, a hallmark of Alzheimer's dementia.

What You Can Do

The best way to avoid damage from alcohol is to stop drinking entirely. Yes, red wine does offer the benefit of resveratrol. This phytonutrient is high in antioxidants and fights inflammation. It also helps moderate blood sugar.

But you can get resveratrol elsewhere, including red grapes and blueberries.

If you can't stop drinking entirely, save your drinking for special occasions, and limit yourself to one small glass. That way you can know you are not hurting your brain.

Whatever you do, strive to drink in moderation.[94]

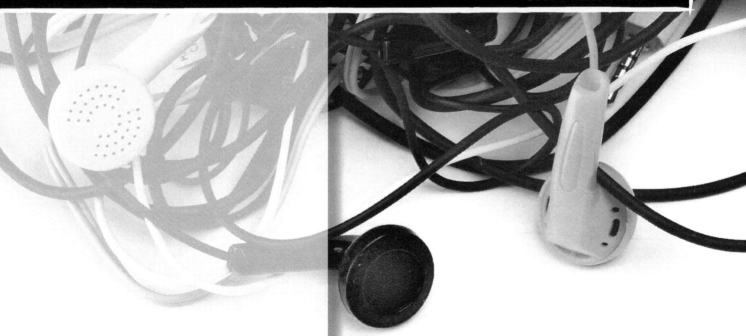

Chapter 15

Rid Your Body of Stress

"I promise you nothing is as chaotic as it seems. Nothing is worth diminishing your health. Nothing is worth poisoning yourself into stress, anxiety, and fear."

- Steve Maraboli

A Tale of Two Parents

Like so many immigrant sons before me, I longed to have my parents join me in the United States. They would be leaving a culture based on family dynamics and close-knit contacts, one in which family members called one another daily and visited often, one with many friends and community relationships.

So I knew they might face a difficult transition.

They came in the winter. I was working long hours as a physician. A language barrier separated them from my American-born wife and from the TV and the radio. We could afford only limited phone calls with friends and family in Iran.

Almost immediately, my mother's interest in her daily routines diminished. As she grew increasingly isolated, I began to notice that her memory was getting worse. Nothing I did seemed to help.

Three days before she was scheduled to go back to Iran, she had a stroke. Thankfully she suffered no significant motor or memory impairment, but after that experience, she has not returned to the U.S. Every time I ask, she refuses.

My father has a stronger spiritual faith. This allowed him to cope better. He intentionally established familiar routines of eating and sleeping, prayer and other activities.

In the spring, he planted a small garden in our backyard. Tending this added sunshine and physical exercise to his routines.

He came to enjoy his visit here in the U.S. and, when the time came, he did not want to go back to Iran.

Two parents. The same stressful situation. Two responses. Two results—one healthy, the other not.

Our Stressful Lives

You also have stress in your life. Most of us do. We wake up after a limited number of hours of interrupted sleep. We rush around getting ready for work and instead of a good breakfast, we grab a piece of pizza from the fridge or skip breakfast entirely.

We begin answering emails or texts as we shave or put on make-up. We yell at the kids to hurry up and then spend frantic minutes searching for car keys.

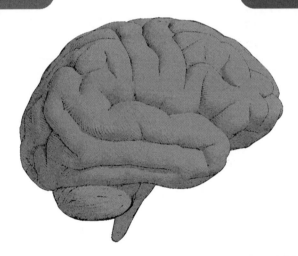

Physical
- Headaches and tense muscles
- Rapid heartbeast
- Diarrhea or constipation
- Nausea and dizziness

Emotional
- Irritability or short temper
- Moodiness
- Often feeling fearful or anxious
- Sense of loneliness

Spiritual
- Reality
- Meaning
- Justice
- Fairness
- Values

Cognitive and Mental
- Inability to concentrate
- Increasing worrying
- Forgetfulness
- Poor judgment

Sources of stress vary significantly from person to person, but we can usually divide stressors into four groups: physical, mental, spiritual and emotional.

In the car, the radio delivers bad news—another shooting spree, a forecast of bad weather, more trouble for the economy.

Work also has its stressors, and when we get home, who has time to relax? Day after day, this stressful routine continues, and we wonder why our health suffers.

What you may not realize is that stress and Alzheimer's are close family members. If we can reduce stress, cognition will improve.

If we don't reduce stress, eventually—and possibly sooner—we will pay the price in impaired cognitive function.

My father found a way to cope with the stressors of living in a new country. Whatever the source of your stress, how you choose to respond can minimize the effects of stress on your life as well.

What is Stress?

Stress begins with a danger, real or perceived. Perhaps you've lost sight of your toddler, an oncoming car has veered into your lane or you realize you might be late to a job interview.

When your body senses danger, your brain sends out an alert that releases a surge of hormones, including adrenaline and cortisol.

The adrenaline signals your heart to beat faster, your brain to receive an extra burst of oxygen and your muscles to get additional blood. The adrenaline also prompts a burst of energy so you can deal with the threat quickly and decisively.

The elevated cortisol turns down systems you don't need, like the digestive and reproductive systems (among others). This gives you extra resources to fight the danger.

In cases of acute stress, the danger goes away. You find your lost toddler, you avoid the oncoming car or you make it to your interview on time. In these cases, acute stress has helped you deal with an immediate threat.

Chronic stress, however, does not go away. Perhaps you have a boss who doesn't appreciate you, overlapping deadlines, an estranged daughter or son or unexpected financial concerns.

With these and other lingering stressors, the adrenaline keeps pumping, the cortisol stays elevated and stress becomes a constant companion. Stress like this makes it hard to control your mood, get jobs done and remember the good in your life. It's extremely hazardous to your health and especially your brain.

Chronic Stress and Your Brain

By now, you know that inflammation, like stress, is an immune response, so it won't surprise you to learn that inflammation and stress operate side by side. Stress signals inflammation, and as long as they both turn off when they are supposed to, everything is okay.

The elevated cortisol that accompanies chronic stress results in the following, all of which increase your risk of Alzheimer's dementia:

- **Weakens the blood-brain barrier,** allowing more germs, heavy metals, harmful chemicals and other toxins into your brain
- **Creates free radicals** that cause oxidation, or "rusting," in the brain
- **Halts production of BDNF,** which slows or halts the creation of new brain cells—especially in the hippocampus, the part of your brain associated with memories
- **Reduces levels of neurotransmitters** (nerve messengers)

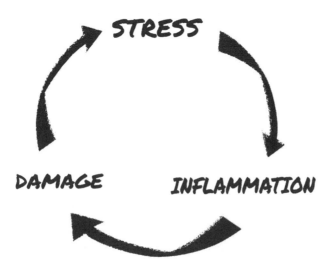

Stress creates a cruel cycle in your body.

How to Reduce Your Stress

The following techniques will help you deal with the stressors in your life that tend to linger:

Increase your sense of control: Regardless of the stressor, you can choose how you respond. This choice will help you gain a sense of control, and your stress will diminish.

Let's say a colleague at work is after your job. This colleague criticizes you publicly and even makes fun of you in meetings. You become angry and extremely anxious about your job. Your stress rises so much that you lose sleep, and this affects your work performance, adding to your anxiety.

Then one day you decide to change your response to the situation. Instead of getting angry and anxious, you begin encouraging this colleague and find opportunities to speak well of her in the presence of your boss.

You ask this colleague for some advice on personal concerns. And in meetings, you ask for her opinion.

None of this is easy, but you are in control. Chances are very good your stress will decrease.

This is my friend's story. Within a month, her tactics had succeeded. The colleague no longer abused their relationship, and my friend could sleep peacefully at night.

High levels of stress + a decision to control what

she could = less stress for my friend and a happier work environment. How can you have more control?

Keep a stress diary: Write down what causes you stress. Then write down as many solutions as you can. This will improve your sense of control.

Exercise: When faced with danger, we have a "fight or flight" response. Chronic stress comes from being unable to do either. Because exercise provides a safe facsimile of the flight response, it will often decrease your cortisol level. This allows you to be calmer. Aerobic exercise is especially good.

Decrease your caffeine and alcohol: Both elevate stress.

Stop smoking: Nicotine is a stimulant.

Meditation: This is so important to your overall cognitive health that I have a separate chapter devoted to it. For now, remember, as long as the meditation takes you out of yourself, out of the time and place you are, and into a place of calm and peace, your stress will decrease.

Try mindful body movement: You can find classes locally or online. Yoga and tai chi are two examples.

Use relaxation techniques: Here's a simple one: First, clench and then relax your feet. Do the same for your knees and work up your body to your shoulders (often tense), your neck and your face. Stay in this relaxed state for up to five minutes.

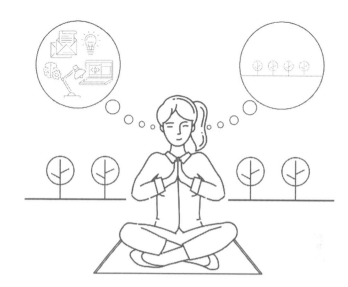

Meditation can decrease stress by taking your mind away from stressors.

Take control of your time: A lot of chronic stress comes from mismanagement of time.

Laugh: Create a list of funny movies guaranteed to make you laugh. Watch funny **YouTube** videos. Try learning a new dance step (in private!). Spend some time with kids.

Spend time with friends or family: You'll want to do this with people you feel safe with, who can calm you down and reassure you.

Volunteer your time and energy in the service of others: This helps get your mind off your worries.

Say no: Some people can't say no because they want others to like them, because they fear rejection or conflict or because they want to feel significant. But scheduling more than you can comfortably handle adds stress to your life. If this is a consistent problem, you might consider counseling. Your brain will thank you!

Other techniques: Pet your pet, hug your loved one, start a gratitude journal, get a massage, drink herbal or black tea or listen to calming music.

The Value of Faith Practices for Your Peace of Mind

There seems to be no doubt that people who engage in religious or spiritual activities as a group are happier and enjoy many physical and emotional benefits, including decreased stress.[95]

This occurs independently of any specific religion, theology or spirituality. It's the faith in something outside ourselves that seems to make the difference for people. We are witnessing science and spirituality coming together.

These benefits extend to cognitive health. Researchers have seen a strong correlation between religious or spiritual activity and lower memory impairment, lower cortisol levels, lower catecholamines and more balanced sugar levels in the blood.

Brain scans show that people with faith practices have similar patterns and connections between neurons, connections that may lead to the health benefits listed above. It all adds up to less stress.

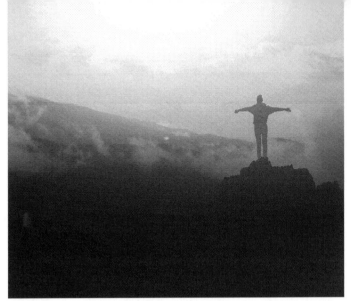

Faith practices can benefit your cognitive health.

Four faith practices that help lower stress

- **Prayer:**
  Brain scans indicate that prayer affects the brain by activating the frontal lobes, resulting in improved attention, mental performance and a corresponding decrease in anxiety.

- **Meditation:**
  I discuss meditation in depth in the next section, because it also contributes to cognitive health and mediates chronic inflammation. Many religions teach meditation as a way to connect more closely to a higher power. For many, meditation ranks with prayer as a religious or spiritual activity.[96]

- **Community:**
  Gather together with others who share your chosen spiritual path. These gatherings, which can take place in synagogues, mosques, churches, temples

or other religious settings, will stimulate your mind and spirit.[97] Yoga gatherings, meditation centers and philosophical book clubs can also provide a meaningful community if they are more aligned with your worldview.

- *Gratitude:*
  Robert A. Emmons, a scientific expert on gratitude, says that it can improve your immune function (thereby helping to decrease chronic inflammation) and reduce the risk of depression and anxiety.[98] I believe it works because it will take your mind off your problems and focus it on the higher power which brings good into your life.[99]

Individuals with a spiritual practice have an inner source of peace. They usually experience less fear and anxiety as a consequence.

Because of this, neuroscience research suggests that religious practices like prayer, meditation, gathering together and gratitude will reduce both your stress and your risk of Alzheimer's.

Chapter 16

Rid Your Mind of Anxious Thoughts

> *"Saying yes to happiness is saying no to things and people that stress you out."*
> -Thema Davis

When I was working nights in an emergency room, I often faced very critical cases, such as gunshot wounds, suicide attempts or the sudden death of an infant.

These cases were physically, emotionally and spiritually distressing. Sometimes it became necessary for me to step outside into the night, look at the stars and breathe deeply, so I could find some peace.

I still rely heavily on meditation for the peace, so I am very pleased to suggest it as a part of your Dementia Action Plan. I have found it incredibly valuable, and I think you will as well.

A Description of Meditation

Stated very simply, meditation is a way to take control of your thoughts. It allows you to take your mind off daily concerns, dismiss harmful thought patterns and pay attention to what will help you.

Rebecca Gladding, who writes often about meditation, describes it as "a mental gym for attention." As in a regular gym, she says, it will take time to strengthen your ability to rest your thoughts. You'll also need to practice every day.[100]

But the benefit for your brain and overall health will be as powerful as the benefits from physical exercise.

Meditation that Helps Your Brain

Often when we feel fear, worry or concern, we respond emotionally and feel out of control. Our thoughts become more and more unsettled and agitated. These disruptive thought patterns add stress to our lives, impede our sleep, disrupt our lives, hinder our relationships and cause problems for our brains.

We need a way to connect these disruptive thoughts to the more analytical portion of our brain rather than to our emotional response system. If we can strengthen the link between our thoughts and our analytical response system, we will be able to deal with our fears and concerns more mindfully and calmly.

The following meditation technique will help you do just that, but be warned: You will need to train your mind to do this, just as you would have to train your body to run a marathon.

At first, it might seem like your brain just can't settle enough to meditate, but keep practicing. It will come.

How to meditate

1. Find a comfortable place to sit. Let your whole body relax, and then focus on your breathing. Feel the breath. Let it become regular.

2. If sounds or discomforts distract you, name each one. Give it your attention for a moment and then set it aside and return to your breathing.

3. If thoughts distract you, accept the thoughts. Let them linger for a moment. Then mindfully set them aside and return to your breathing. Some will be worries or concerns. Acknowledge these concerns. Then set them aside, and return to your breathing.

4. Do the same with emotions. Accept the emotion and name it. Feel its every effect on your body. Then set it aside and return to your breathing.

5. Be gentle on these thoughts and emotions. Give them their moment. They do not control you. You don't have to be afraid. Then let them go.

For more information and instruction on this technique, please refer to the free guided meditation entitled "Complete Meditation Instructions" offered by the UCLA Mindful Awareness Research Center.[101]

How Meditation Helps Your Brain

Meditation decreases stress:

Sometimes it's hard to figure out exactly what in your life is causing stress. A generalized stress seems to be always present, more as a habit than from any one cause.

Meditation is one of the best ways to relieve this generalized stress. Instead of kicking your immune system into high gear and triggering your flight-or-fight response, meditation helps you stay calm.

And if your meditation is part of your religious observation, it can help remind you of a higher power's goodness and ultimate control, a powerful boost to peace.

Meditation increases your Brain-Derived Neurotrophic Factor (BDNF):

For your cognitive health, perhaps the most crucial benefit of meditation is its ability to increase BDNF in the brain.

To review, BDNF is a protein that produces and protects neurons in your brain and central nervous system.

In 2017, researchers at the University of Southern California measured the BDNF levels of 38 people before and after a three-month meditation retreat. The result: Those who meditated increased their BDNF levels by 280%.[102]

The theory is that meditation:

- Causes anatomical improvements in the brain
- Creates new circles and connections between neurons and neurogenesis

- Enhances memory
- Decreases neurodegenerative disease

BDNF is a powerful tool for preserving the health of your brain. This makes meditation very important.

Meditation enlarges the gray matter in your brain:

The gray matter in your brain is made up mostly of neurons. When you lose gray matter, you're losing neurons. Having fewer neurons affects your memory and cognitive abilities. Meditation can halt that decline.

A study at Harvard involved 16 people who took an eight-week mindfulness course with guided meditations. Progressive MRI scans showed larger and larger concentrations of gray matter.

Other studies have shown that meditation can result in larger hippocampal and frontal volumes of gray matter.[103] The hippocampus, remember, is the region of the brain involved in learning and memory. So meditation can powerfully reduce your risk of dementia.

Meditation improves your emotional health:

Meditation improves your ability to concentrate on healthy thoughts rather than anxious, angry and disruptive thoughts. This increases your self-awareness, imagination and creativity. It also develops your patience and tolerance of other people.

Ultimately you become less critical of yourself, happier and more optimistic.[104]

Meditation improves chronic health conditions:

By making you calmer, meditation helps you manage the symptoms of asthma, chronic pain, heart disease, high blood pressure, irritable bowel syndrome, sleep problems and tension headaches.

It also helps to decrease inflammation, balance sugar levels, improve cardiovascular and GI function, speed up your metabolism and may even address the underlying causes of cancer.

Meditation can't necessarily replace traditional medical treatment, however, so follow your doctor's instructions for treating your chronic diseases.

Even so, along with exercise, meditation can dramatically improve your health.

Some Things to Consider

Adapt meditation that fits into your worldview, religion or practice of spirituality

The method I have described can be adapted to your own belief system. If you are on a secular path, this meditation does not have to include the concept of a higher being.

If you are a person of faith, you can include God in whatever way you see fit.

A Christian friend relates the emphasis on breathing to the Christian Holy Spirit, who is often called the "breath of God." She says being aware of his constant presence helps her set aside her concerns more effectively.

Find a way to adapt the technique to whatever path your are on.

Choose a time that fits your lifestyle:

I believe that consistency helps, just as it does with physical exercise. It helps to set a time limit for your meditation. This limit makes the practice more intentional and easier to sustain.

I meditate every morning for 45 minutes. At the end of this time, I feel noticeably calmer, and I am in better control of my thoughts. If you are new to meditation, however, I would recommend starting with ten minutes and going on from there.

Throughout the day, you might find yourself taking only a few minutes to meditate so that as you mindfully breathe you can set aside particularly troubling thoughts. I have been known to try this at stoplights, for just 30 seconds. It helps!

Choose a place that works for you

It's nice to think of having a "room of your own" for meditation, but all you really need is a quiet place where you won't be interrupted. (And if you are, welcome the interruption, then set it aside, and return to your breathing!)

Meditating in nature has a proven calming effect on our bodies. In Japan, this is called **Shinrin-Yoku**, a term that means "forest bathing." It can refer to meditation that takes place in any natural environment.

The practice offers so many wellness benefits that parks throughout the world now offer Shinrin-Yoku therapy walks with guided activities and meditations.[105]

These activities and meditations may not be available to you, but you can certainly take a walk yourself without guidance from anyone. Go slowly, breathe deeply and focus your thoughts on the nature around you.

Consider guided imagery

One of the best ways to calm your mind is through guided imagery, which you can do with an instructor or with the help of free online downloads.[106] You can easily find options that match your philosophy or spiritual beliefs.

Chapter 17

Rid Your Body and Mind of Tension

"Nurturing yourself is not selfish — it is essential to your survival and well-being."

-Renee Peterson Trudeau

In the emergency department, we often use physical touch to calm an anxious patient. Physical touch affects the severity of their disease, how long they stay in the hospital and their long-term outcome.

If a patient comes in who is having a heart attack, for example, we follow a standard protocol of oxygen, aspirin and cardiac catheterization. We also provide the simple touch of reassurance.

We know the body will respond to this calming physical touch.

In the table below, I review some of the ways you can receive physical stimulation to improve your health.

Some of these interventions have proven benefits: massage, music therapy and biofeedback, for example. Others have mixed evidence regarding benefits, and for a few, there are no proven benefits (yet).

However, because they are a safe and non-invasive technique, I believe they are worth trying if only to gauge their effectiveness for yourself. You may find them extremely helpful, especially in relieving stress.

TABLE: Techniques of Physical Stimulation, Description and Benefits

Technique	Process	Benefits
Acupuncture	A treatment in which specific points on the body are stimulated, most often using needles on the skin	Used primarily to relieve pain; also fatigue, GI problems and thyroid function; thought to improve cognitive function
Craniosacral Therapy (CST)	A therapy used to apply massage to the scalp, spinal column, and sacrum	Thought to improve the brain's glymphatic system, which removes waste from the brain; restores bones to natural positions; relieves stress

Technique	Process	Benefits
Spinal Manipulation	A treatment that involves moving the joints in the spine, massage, exercise and physical therapy	Provides feedback to the brain, which helps with back and neck pain as well as improving the GI, endocrine, cardiovascular and respiratory systems
Music therapy	People listen to or play music.	Decreases stress, PTSD, pain; stimulates the mind to remember and imagine
Massage	A technique whereby muscles and joints are manipulated to enhance health and well-being	Relieves stress, tension, depression, headaches or other pain; can accompany meditation; helps to restore normal circulation, reducing inflammation; enhances healing
Aromatherapy and Massage	They involve using essential oils to promote health, relaxation, sleep and other beneficial aspects of life; often accompanied by massage.	Used as a non-pharmacological intervention to stimulate neurons and manage conditions associated with Alzheimer's such as agitation, depression, insomnia and cognitive decline. Aromas can act as antioxidants; by stimulating olfactory nerves, aromatherapy stimulates the limbic system, amygdala and hippocampus in the brain, improving nerve function

Technique	Process	Benefits
Micro-Current Therapy	A very low current is passed through affected cells and tissue to stimulate healing.	Enhances function, improves the body's chemical balance, optimizes mitochondria, connects nerve branches to improve neural communication
Cranial Electrical Stimulation	A battery-operated, noninvasive device delivers a low level of electrical current to the head.	Reduces sleep and mood disturbances; increases blood flow and the levels of neurotransmitters in the cerebrospinal fluid—including endorphins, the feel-good hormone
Pulsed Electromagnetic Fields Therapy[107]	Tubes placed on the body receive a magnetic field that penetrates cells and stimulates chemical and electrical processes.	Thought to enhance energy at the cellular level, decrease inflammation, speed healing and alleviate pain; in the brain, stimulates receptors and neurons, improving function and stabilizing cell membranes; can also reduce oxidative stress; may even improve cognitive impairment in people with Alzheimer's dementia

Chapter 18

Rid Your Body of Gut Problems

> *"All disease begins in the gut."*
> — *Hippocrates*

"You are what you eat." I'm sure you've heard that.

Let's be more precise.

You are what you eat and digest and absorb. Your gastrointestinal system (or GI) is responsible for all of these processes. This chapter is about how you can best encourage your GI to work on behalf of your brain.

Throughout this chapter, I will use the word **gut**. By this, I mean your entire digestive system, starting with your mouth and extending to the end of your intestines.[108]

Your gut runs through your body, but it is also open to the environment, including the air, water and food you bring into your body.

This introduces into your gut a mix of microorganisms called a *microbiome*. This mix is unique to you. It includes bacteria, fungus, parasites and even viruses.

In many ways, your health depends on this unique mix. If your microbiome has a proper balance, you will live a comfortable, healthy life.

For too long, we have undervalued the health of the gut. It can improve your life and especially your brain.

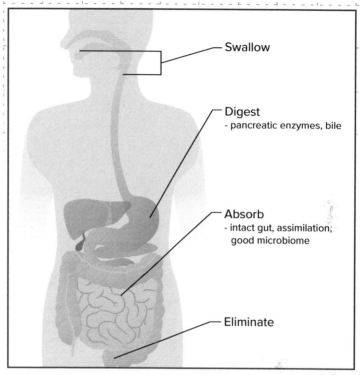

Your gut includes your entire digestive system, from your mouth to the end of your intestines.

The Importance of Your Gut— Let Me Count the Ways

1. *Your gut has a dedicated system of nerves*: Your gut is so essential to your cognitive health that your body provides an elaborate and exclusive network of nerves between your brain and your gut. This makes it easy for your gut to communicate with your brain. You experience this close communication between your brain and your gut when worries or anxieties trigger diarrhea or nausea.

2. ***Your gut has 50% of your body's neurotransmitters:*** These transport messages across the synaptic spaces between neurons. Remarkably, your GI tract contains more than 50% of your body's neurotransmitters,[109] some of which originate in the gut. That's a lot of brain power invested in your digestive system.

3. ***Your gut has many, many immune functions***: Your gut performs drastically more immune functions than the rest of your body. And as I'm sure you know by now, when the immune system gets involved, the potential for chronic inflammation increases. This means the gut has a lot to say about how much inflammation occurs in your brain.

   Bottom line: Your gut is very important to cognitive health.

The Sequence of Digestion

Digestion starts when you first smell or see food and proceeds step-by-step through your body until you eliminate waste. In between, your body needs the correct enzymes, acids and bacteria for optimal digestion.

In a healthy gut, everything operates very smoothly. You chew up the food. It goes to the stomach where fatty acids and bile from the pancreas and gall bladder continue the digestion. Because of this, when the food reaches the intestines, it can be absorbed into your body and put to use.

If any part of this sequence is impaired, your health suffers.

Gut Health in the Upper GI Tract

Your food can sometimes go through to your intestines without being ready to be absorbed. When this happens, the food can severely damage your intestines.

Why the Upper Gut Sometimes Fails to Prepare Food for the Intestines

- Too much sugar
- Harmful bacteria in your mouth
- Inadequate chewing
- Toxins
- Allergies
- Anxiety
- Age
- Too little acid in your stomach
- Too much acid in your stomach
- Thyroid problems
- Using high heat when cooking
- Insufficient enzymes

How to Improve Your Upper Gut Health

- *Chew your food thoroughly:* Your saliva begins preparing your food to be absorbed. If you rush your chewing, you'll miss an essential step.

- *Eat lots of vegetables and anti-inflammatory foods:* These prebiotic foods encourage the good bacteria throughout your gut, including the upper GI tract.

- *Limit sugar in your diet:* Sugar encourages harmful bacteria to thrive, choking out the good bacteria. Sugar causes trouble at every step of your digestive tract, so you'll read this advice several times in this chapter. It's important information.

- *Talk with your doctor if you experience symptoms of "acid/upset stomach":* The symptoms of low acid and high acid are very similar. You need to know which you are experiencing so you can treat the problem correctly. Acid protects your gut by killing harmful bacteria, so low acid can be a serious problem.

- *Include raw foods in your diet and hydrate 20 minutes before meals* to improve enzyme efficiency.

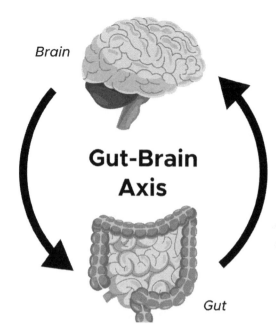

The health of your gut determines the health of your brain.

Gut Health in the Intestines

Now we get to the place where your food can be absorbed: your intestines. There are two critical requirements for optimizing your intestinal function:

1. *A healthy intestinal surface:* The surface of your intestines should serve as a gatekeeper that allows the proper nutrients and molecules to transfer from your intestines into your bloodstream. At the same time, this intestinal surface needs to keep other items inside the gut. Some of these items that are kept inside the intestines will be used to maintain a healthy microbiome. The rest will be discharged as waste.

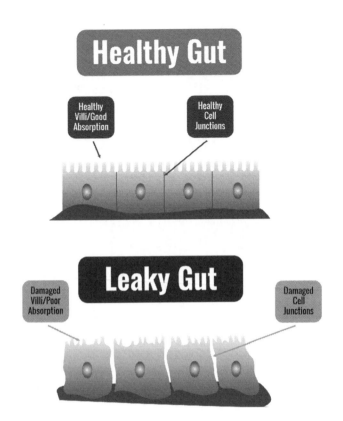

A healthy gut serves as a gatekeeper. A leaky gut allows too much in and out of the intestinal wall.

2. ***Healthy bacteria:*** The second critical requirement for optimizing digestive function is to provide everything that healthy microbes need to thrive in your intestines. These healthy organisms improve digestion, strengthen your immune system and support health throughout your body, including your brain. Keeping the good microorganisms healthy is crucial. Otherwise, you will experience microbiome imbalance.

Intestinal Problem #1: Leaky Gut

The surface of your intestines has ***tight junctions*** that link the surface cells. During healthy digestion, these tight junctions stay closed, allowing only properly digested nutrients to pass from the intestines into the bloodstream.

When tight junctions aren't working properly, the surface of the intestine becomes more permeable. We call this *intestinal permeability,* or a "leaky gut."

With a leaky gut, undigested food particles, toxins, yeast and other pathogens can go in and out of the intestines. Your intestinal microbiome suffers because it needs some of these particles to thrive. Your health suffers when the toxins leak through!

When these particles enter the tissues outside your intestines, your liver tries to screen out the intruders but soon gets behind. Your immune system then gets involved, which causes inflammation and results in a full-fledged war between your body and the invaders.

And like any war, there's a lot of collateral damage.

Unfortunately, the standard American diet (SAD) and our typical lifestyle make it extremely hard for the tight junctions to function correctly.

Symptoms of a leaky gut

- Chronic diarrhea, constipation, gas or bloating
- Headaches
- Excessive fatigue

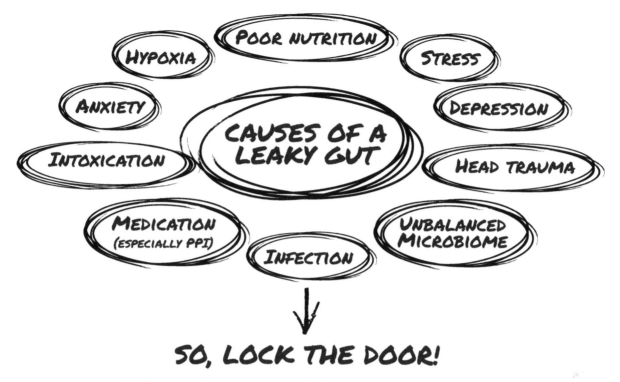

SO, LOCK THE DOOR!

With your choices, you can help protect your intestines.

- Skin rashes and other conditions such as acne, eczema or rosacea
- Cravings for sugar or carbs
- Arthritis or joint pain
- Depression, anxiety, ADD or ADHD
- Brain fog and memory loss[110]

If you do have leaky gut, what begins as a fairly common symptom (headache, constipation, etc.) can lead to serious chronic illnesses such as arthritis, lupus, celiac disease and possibly even Alzheimer's dementia.

Leaky Gut and the Brain

A leaky gut almost inevitably affects your cognition because of the inflammation that occurs in response. If your immune system successfully removes the danger, that's okay—this is a case of acute inflammation.

But if the battle against the threat continues, the inflammation becomes chronic. With so many neurons traveling between the gut and the brain, they get caught in the crossfire of chronic inflammation, and your cognition suffers.

What You Can Do to Fix a Leaky Gut

1. *Eat more fiber:* This protects against gut permeability by maintaining a healthy mucus layer in the gut. Get both soluble fiber, which keeps digestion moving, and insoluble fiber, which keeps your stools from becoming too watery. Opt for the fiber found in vegetables and whole grains rather than the refined fiber found in processed foods.[111]

2. *Be careful with lectins:* You can find these proteins in raw legumes and grains, dairy products and some vegetables. They resist digestion and often go through the upper GI without being broken down enough, allowing them to run right over the tight junctions in your intestine. This contributes to leaky gut. Our bodies recognize these lectins as a threat, and immune cells react against them. As a result, some people develop allergies and sensitivities to lectins. Legumes that have been soaked and boiled have much lower levels of lectins. Sprouted grains also have lower levels, as do fermented foods with lectins. Many of these foods are a fantastic source of vitamins, minerals, vegetable protein and phytonutrients, so process carefully and then eat and enjoy to your health.

3. *Deal with food allergies:* These activate an inflammatory immune response and start a cascade of reactions. If you don't address these food allergies and sensitivities, chronic inflammation will occur in the lining of the intestines, affecting absorption and creating a leaky gut. Seek out your doctor's advice or consult with a nutrition expert if you suspect food allergies. Along with scheduling blood tests, this professional may want you to keep a food diary to record your body's responses to food.

4. *Test your gluten sensitivity/allergy:* Gluten is a natural substance found in wheat and other similar grains such as rye, barley and oats. Not everyone has an allergy or sensitivity to gluten, but for those who do, gluten will contribute to leaky gut and chronic inflammation. It's worth checking out!

5. *Avoid sugar:* Sugar feeds a yeast overgrowth to which your body reacts, leading your immune response to trigger inflammation. To counteract this, avoid all kinds of sugar, including corn syrup, molasses, high fructose corn syrup, brown sugar and cane sugar. My advice: When the craving for sugar hits, eat a quarter cup of nuts. The fat in the nuts can help quench the sugar craving.

6. *Avoid the four white demons:* White bread, white rice, white pasta and white potatoes break down quickly into sugar and feed the yeast in your gut. The fiber in whole grains slows down the sugar absorption.

7. *Eat more vegetables and low-sugar fruits:* These are good for everything else in your body. Add your gut to the list!

8. *Avoid alcohol:* Alcohol is a toxin. It irritates the gut.

Intestinal Problem #2: Microbiome Imbalance, or Dysbiosis

Your microbiome is a complex ecosystem that contains more than 38 trillion bacterial cells.[112] When food, toxins, medication or lifestyle choices alter this ecosystem, microbiome imbalance (also known as *dysbiosis*) results. This is a serious problem for your overall health and well-being.

What Causes Microbiome Imbalance?

Anything that affects your overall microbiome can create microbiome imbalance in your intestines. This includes your heredity, where you live, your lifestyle choices, what you eat, your stress level, social interactions and sense of well-being, as well as the environmental toxins you encounter in your daily life.

The Overuse of Antibiotics

Our whole body including the skin, nose, mouth, lungs and our GI system—is home to trillions of healthy bacteria that are important to our metabolism and immunity. This includes our large and small intestines.

Antibiotics, which you take to destroy harmful bacteria, also destroy these beneficial bacteria. So any antibiotic use poses a risk to your gut microbiome.

Our medical system relies heavily on antibiotics, and that can be a problem for our collective gut.

But the way we raise our livestock also relies heavily on antibiotics. Beef, chicken and many other animal sources contain antibiotics, antifungals and antiprotozoals.

All of these contribute to microbiome imbalance.

Stress

Your level of stress has an almost immediate impact on your GI tract. Are you nervous? Here comes diarrhea or nausea. Anxious? Bloating and stomach cramps. Agitated? Constipation or indigestion.

When your body senses a situation where you need to either fight or flee from danger, your sympathetic system kicks into gear. You can think of this as your "flight or fight" response.

It closes down openings called sphincters all along your GI tract. Blood vessels also contract, inhibiting the ability of GI secretions to have their desired effect. The intestinal muscles that usually mix and move contents through your GI tract also shut down.

This gives you the energy and strength to deal with the immediate danger. When the danger ends, your body switches back to a parasympathetic response. Think of this as your "rest and digest" response.

This response slows your heart rate, relaxes sphincters in your gut, increases secretions and keeps the contractions that mix and move contents through the GI tract working smoothly.

The real damage occurs when there is no sudden danger, just a lingering sense of things not being right. Your body responds with the fight or flee impulse, but because it's not real, this danger never goes away.

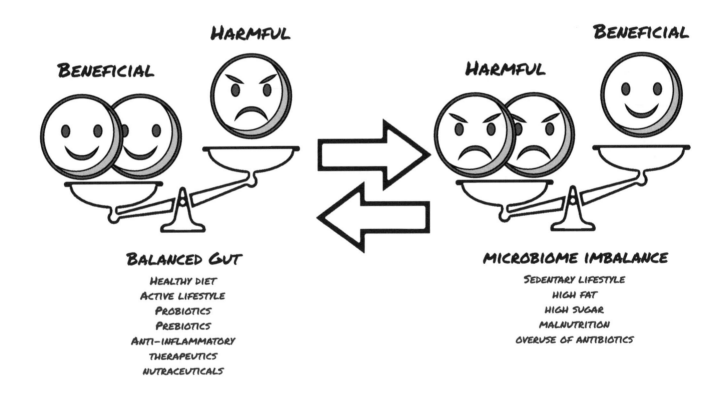

An overview of microbiome gut imbalance

The result of this chronic stress? Spasms in your esophagus, stomach discomfort, nausea, diarrhea or constipation that lingers and lasts and becomes habitual. Your entire gut, and especially your intestines, suffer damage. So whatever else you do to improve your gut—and I hope you'll do plenty—remember to work on your stress levels.

What You Can Do to Fix Your Microbiome Imbalance

Besides being careful with the use of antibiotics and limiting stress, you can:

- *Cut out added sugar*: One more time: Sugar feeds harmful bacteria. Less sugar in your gut contributes to better cognitive functioning.[113]
- *Talk to your doctor about a probiotic*
- *Try fermented foods*: These include sauerkraut, kimchi, kefir and unsweetened yogurt.
- *Limit processed foods*: These are high in added sugars and unhealthy fats.
- *Choose healthy fats*: See the section on fats in the nutrition chapter.
- *Eat a high-fiber diet*: Include both soluble and insoluble fiber.
- *Limit red meat and animal products*: Studies have shown that a high-meat diet increases the gut bacteria that cause inflammation.[114]
- *Stay hydrated*: This helps digestion and keeps stools moving through the colon.

- *Exercise*: This guards against constipation and helps you maintain a healthy weight.
- *Get enough B-complex vitamins, calcium, magnesium, beta-carotene and zinc*: See Chapter 12 for more on nutritional gaps and supplements.
- *Get a little dirty*: We need some of the bacteria that live in a non-sterile world. For example, children growing up with a dog develop fewer allergies. Also, the good clean dirt we encounter while gardening boosts our immune system. So stop using antibacterial soaps because they destroy all bacteria, even the ones we need.[115]

There's Hope!

I find the close connection between the gut and the brain very encouraging. It offers so many ways to limit your risk of Alzheimer's.

In my journey back to health, I started by limiting stress, eliminating tobacco and improving my nutrition. All these steps had a significant impact on gut health, and I think now that's why these steps made such a difference in my health.

So calm down. Eliminate toxins. Eat food that is good for you. This will improve your gut health.

And then, enjoy your improved gut health!

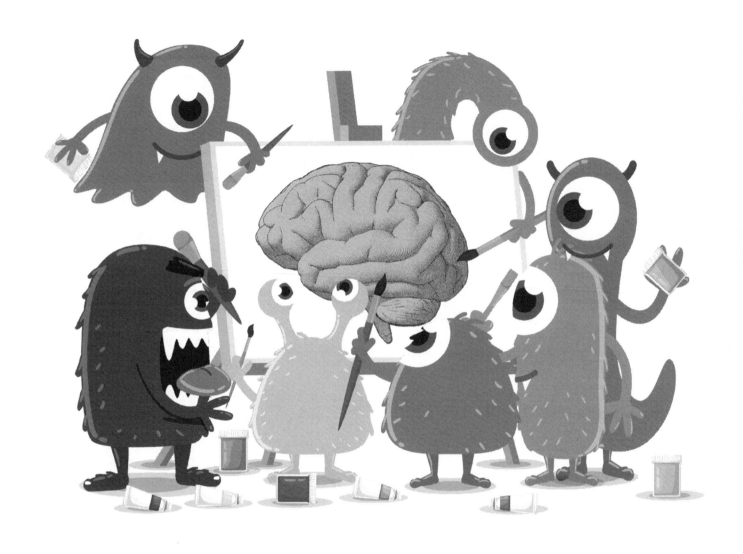

Healthy and plentiful gut bacteria will paint a healthy picture of your brain!

Chapter 19

Rid Your Body of Toxins

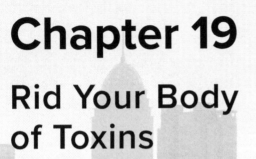

Prime your tissues to combat environmental toxins.

Maybe you are what you eat, but you are also what you breathe, touch and drink.

Unfortunately, our modern environment holds many threats to our well-being. In this chapter, I will describe the threats that exist around you, including toxins, pesticides, personal care products and other dangers. I will also describe how they affect your body, and then suggest ways that you can limit these threats.

As you read this chapter on toxins, you may wonder how we manage to survive, but we are fortunate that the human body is well equipped to do battle against these threats, especially if you help by making lifestyle changes.

The Damage Toxins Do

1. *Toxins damage the nervous system*, leading to the following:

   - *Learning and behavioral disabilities*
   - *Psychological problems*
   - *Brain dysfunction* that includes a decreased ability to concentrate, problem-solving, memory and learning deficits

2. *Toxins damage the immune system:*
   If your immune system has to deal with too many environmental toxins, it becomes weaker, resulting in chronic inflammation, oxidative stress and eventually chronic diseases.

3. *Toxins damage mitochondria:*
   Mitochondria are specialized structures in the cell that produce energy (see Chapter 8). Because of their fat content, mitochondria tend to store toxins, leading to unnatural cell death.

4. *Toxins damage hormones:*
   Some toxins increase or decrease normal hormone levels, mimic hormones and alter the production of hormones. They also interfere with hormonal signaling, compete for essential nutrients and accumulate in the organs that produce hormones. You will learn more about hormones in the next chapter.

5. *Toxins damage the genetic material in a cell (RNA, DNA):*
   Your genes are affected by your daily exposure to toxins, causing mutations in cells throughout your body, including the kind that lead to cancer.

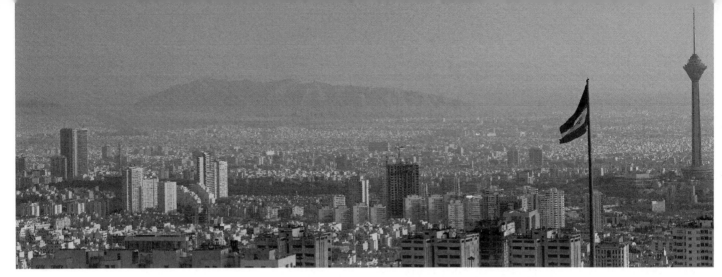

Visible smog in Tehran, Iran, my original home.[118]

This chapter will describe how you can limit your exposure to these environmental toxins and thereby counteract this damage.

Air Pollution

There is strong evidence that air pollution dramatically increases your risk of Alzheimer's disease.

In a 2012 study, exposure to air pollution led to lower scores on cognitive tests, and living close to a high-traffic area has also been associated with smaller brain volume and a decrease in the white matter in the brain that connects different brain regions.[116]

Air pollution is (1) a mixture of solid particles and gases in the air, (2) introduced into the atmosphere by people and (3) threatens living things and the environment.[117]

It can be visible or invisible. The most visible form is smog, as seen in the image above of Tehran, Iran,

considered one of the most densely polluted cities in the world and my original home.

Outside your home: You can breathe in pollution from traffic fumes, power plants, refineries, livestock, wood-burning fireplaces, burning leaves and natural sources like wind-blown dust and wildfires.

Inside your home: You can breathe in carbon monoxide and radon, fumes from cleaners and other household chemicals, mold and pollen, dust mites and chemicals like formaldehyde used in the manufacturing of building materials.

How Air Pollution Affects the Brain

Directly : Particles of air pollution travel through the nose or the lining of the nasal passages into the brain. Their presence in the brain triggers an immune response. With sustained pollution exposure, chronic inflammation and all its collateral damage can result.

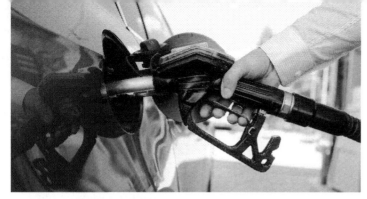

The gasoline burned in cars is a major source of air pollution.

Indirectly: Breathing in air pollution can inflame the lungs, which causes the release of substances like interferon, interleukin, growth factors and other biological compounds that harm the brain and cause inflammation.

Your body can handle larger particles in the air, either by coughing or by sending immune cells called macrophages to engulf the invading particles.

Your body has more trouble with tiny particles—called PM2.5—because these can go through the lung wall and end up in your bloodstream.

Once there, they can circulate to the brain, where they are small enough to pass through the all-important blood-brain barrier.[119]

Three components of air pollution—ozone, nitrogen oxides and PM2.5—may also contribute to problems in the brain because these components create free radicals (oxidative problems) and promote inflammation.

How to Limit the Effects of Air Pollution

In a way, the studies on the connection between air pollution and Alzheimer's are an exciting development. If we can demonstrate conclusively that air pollution causes Alzheimer's, we may be able to lower the incidence of the disease.

In the meantime, here's what you can do to limit your exposure to air pollution:

- *Check your air quality:* Go to our website, InteractWellCare.com, to discover current ozone and particulate matter levels in your location.
- *Purchase a portable or central air cleaning system:* Use a high-quality HEPA filter. Avoid filters using ozone.
- *Stay indoors* if you live near high-traffic areas. Save outdoor activities for early in the day when pollution levels are lower or for days when air pollution levels remain low.
- *Do outdoor workouts in the morning:* Ozone levels are lower at this time of day.
- *Avoid heavy traffic if at all possible:* If you find yourself sitting in traffic, set your fan to recirculate so that you are not drawing in polluted air from outside.
- *Don't smoke (at all)* and especially not indoors.

- **Don't build fires** in your fireplace or wood-burning stove.
- **Avoid burning leaves, trash or other materials.**
- **Avoid using gas-powered lawn or garden equipment** (especially when particulate levels are high).
- **Plant trees, bushes and other greenery outside and include some plants inside**: These filter nitrogen dioxide and particulate matter out of the air.[120]

As I mentioned before, Alzheimer's is often considered an environmental or industrial disease. By limiting your exposure to air pollution, you can take a critical preemptive step toward reducing your risk of cognitive damage.

Pesticides

The term pesticide refers to a broad class of chemical killing agents. They are toxins specifically designed to kill living things.

They serve a purpose by protecting crops and increasing the world's food production. They also protect our homes and workplaces from infestations of cockroaches, rats and other pests.

However, their use permeates every part of our lives—homes, schools, workplaces, parks, swimming pools and forests. Anywhere there are people, there are probably pesticides as well.

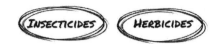
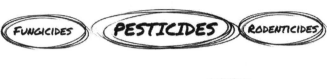
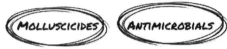

Six kinds of pesticides, all designed to kill living things

Worldwide, pesticide use adds up to approximately 5.6 billion pounds each year. In the United States, we produce over 1 billion pounds of pesticides annually and use more than 350 different pesticides in our homes, buildings, parks, and croplands.

After use, pesticides get recycled in our soil and water, where they continue to do damage. Up to 50 million people in the U.S. obtain their drinking water from groundwater, which is where pesticide contamination is likely to occur.

No wonder humans experience so much damage from pesticides, not just in the United States but around the world as well. According to the World Health Organization, three million cases of pesticide poisoning occur each year, causing more than 200,000 deaths.[121]

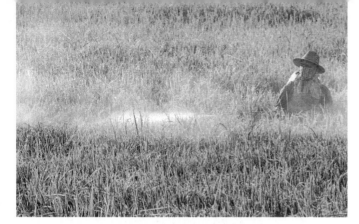

Pesticides present a particular danger to communities near agriculture.

How Pesticides Damage Your Body

Pesticides cause cancer. They also have chemicals that mimic compounds like estrogen, leading to the disruption of normal hormone function. Exposure to pesticides is further associated with earlier onset of puberty, abnormal menstrual cycles and hormonal imbalance.

Many consequences are permanent, affecting not only our bodies but the bodies of our offspring for generations to come. The news for your brain is just as bad.

How Pesticides Damage Your Brain

Pesticides damage us by poisoning nerve tissue either in the brain or spinal cord. Working as an emergency room doctor in an agricultural area, I have encountered this personally. As farmers apply pesticides during certain seasonal periods, I see more patients than usual complaining of headaches, dizziness, nausea, vomiting, sweating, diarrhea and salivation problems. All of these are associated with pesticide exposure.

Chronic exposure, year after year, has been associated with significant cognitive and psychomotor impairment, and even multi-organ failure, which causes your whole body to shut down. Several studies have found a strong association between occupational pesticide exposure and a higher incidence of neurodegenerative diseases such as Parkinson's and Alzheimer's disease.[122]

The world took the first step in seeking to limit human exposure to pesticides in 1995. The United Nations called for a global response to what they called "Persistent Organic Pollutants" (POPs). According to the European Commission on the environment, POPs are "chemical substances that persist in the environment, bioaccumulate through the food web and pose a risk of causing adverse effects to human health and the environment."[123]

Widespread production of this class of pesticides began less than 60 years ago, but there are already detectable levels of POPs found in the tissue of all living things on earth. The dangers they pose:

- POPs have a high potential for accumulating in the food chain.
- They can be transferred widely throughout the environment.
- They are stored in body fat and interfere with standard detoxification systems in the body.

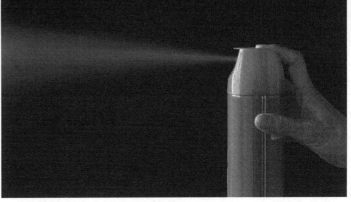

Whatever you spray into the air can end up in your body and brain. Avoid toxic insecticides.

- They harm our immune systems, livers, endocrine system, neurological system and development.
- They have the potential to cause cancer.

In response to the United Nations' mandate, the Stockholm Convention ratified a treaty in 2001 that banned or severely restricted twelve of the most dangerous POPs, and hundreds of countries signed it.

Sadly, the United States has not ratified this treaty, and it seems unlikely ever to do so. Instead, we must take steps as individuals to limit their effects on our lives.

Limiting pesticides in your life is a big job. To simplify things (slightly!), I will discuss each of the six kinds of pesticides separately.

Insecticides, which kill insects

Common forms include mothballs, boric acid and the widely available spray and liquid products you can purchase at the grocery store.

Try to limit these pesticides both in your home and in your yard and garden.

In your home:

- Keep a clean kitchen
- Store non-perishable foods and staples in sealed containers
- Store perishable food, including fruit, in the refrigerator
- Take out the garbage daily
- Wash indoor pets' bedding once a week
- Fix leaky pipes and faucets since damp conditions encourage pests to breed
- Use mousetraps, fly swatters, jar traps and other nontoxic weapons
- As a last resort, hire a licensed extermination service certified by EcoWise, GreenPro, Green Shield or other reputable programs

In your gardens:

- Look into plants that repel insects, like marigolds or pungent basil.
- Put strips of aluminum foil under plants to confuse insects
- Make a solution of one tablespoon of dishwashing soap (minimal dyes or fragrances) with 6 cups of water, and spray this on your plants

Herbicides, which kill weeds

Roundup,® also known as glyphosate, is the most widely used weed killer in the United States. It poses risks for human health. AAtrex (atrazine) is also widely used and can also be hazardous. Even though the EPA decided not to limit its sale, some countries have banned atrazine.

The problem with herbicides for humans comes from drift. Since most herbicides are in spray form, once dispensed, they frequently drift away from the targeted weed into the air we breathe or the produce we grow in our gardens.

In your gardens and lawns:

- Practice weed exclusion when you plant, using weed-free seeds and plants. Use clean equipment and containers.
- Ensure potting materials that are weed-free.
- Pull the weeds by hand or with weeding tools. By rule, you need to get rid of weeds as soon as you see them—"a pull in time saves nine."
- Mulch to discourage weeds
- In a pinch, purchase organic vinegar-based weed killers

Fungicides, which kill fungus

If you have mold in your house, seek professional help. It's a serious threat to your health.

When mildew or some other fungus attacks your vegetable garden, you need a safe form of intervention. Unfortunately, many chemical fungicides are sulfur based and can be irritating to skin and eyes in humans. Breathing in the spray or dust can also cause throat irritation, sneezing and coughing.

Longer-term exposure has led to increased anxiety in animal test subjects, leading to hormonal imbalances and changes in behavior.

Fortunately, there are alternatives.[124] You could use instead:

- *Diluted milk:* Regularly applied to plants, this can reduce mildew and mold by up to 90%. Make a mixture of one part skim milk and nine parts water, and spray it on your plants.
- *Baking soda* also limits fungus. Make a mixture of four teaspoons baking soda, one teaspoon dishwashing soap, and one gallon of water. Spray this on both sides of the leaves.

Rodenticides, which kill rodents

These chemicals kill mice, rats, squirrels, chipmunks, porcupines and other rodents. Many are anticoagulants that work by stopping normal blood clotting.

Yes, we do hate mice and rats.

Yes, we do want to rid our homes of these pests.

But using these toxic killers is a risky solution. Not only are these chemicals potentially toxic to humans, but they are also harmful to any species that encounters them, including our pets who eat the dead rodents.

You can learn more about risks for children, pets and wildlife at the Safe Rodent Control Resource Center website (SafeRodentControl.org).

To limit the use of rodenticides in your home:

- Seal entry points.
- Store food where mice and rats cannot reach it. They won't stay if you don't feed them!
- Keep food spaces clean.
- Remove nesting materials like shredded paper or fabrics.
- Use old-fashioned traps to catch rodents. If you plan to use live traps, check local regulations regarding the release of rodents into the wild.

Molluscicides, which kill slugs and snails:

People generally apply these chemicals as pellets in their gardens. The greatest immediate danger is accidental poisoning of pets, birds and other wildlife.

But there's also a risk from long-term use and exposure, both for you, if you are the gardener, and for the soil and water.

To limit the use of molluscicides in your garden:

- Plant some aromatic herbs like lavender, rosemary and thyme in your garden. Slugs don't like them.
- Increase space between the plants to allow the sun to reach the soil and air to circulate.
- Cut off the bottom of your gallon milk jugs and put them over young plants, which is one of the best non-toxic barriers to slugs. You can remove them once the plant has grown.
- You can also pluck off the slugs by hand.

Antimicrobials, which kill germs

Putting chemicals into products to kill germs is a huge business. Manufacturers put them in soap, detergents, hand wipes, toothpaste, cosmetics, cutting boards, mattress pads and many other products.

But many health experts believe the antimicrobial agents in these products do more harm than good.

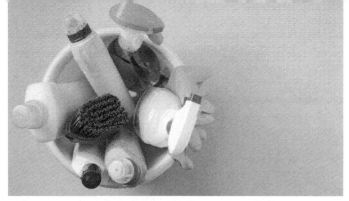

Choose your cleaning products carefully to avoid hurting your health and your family's.

People with prolonged antimicrobial exposure have a higher chance of developing allergies. Your immune system needs some exposure to microbes.

Their widespread use is helping to create antibiotic-resistant bacteria, which threaten your ability to fight life-threatening infections. They can disrupt your body's use of hormones

The antimicrobial agents often end up in your water supply, which has a terrible effect on marine life. *The solution is simple:* Avoid buying antibacterial products.

To limit your use of antimicrobial products:

- Diligently wash your hands using soap and water.

- A good rule of thumb is to wash long enough to sing "Happy Birthday" through twice. That should take 20 seconds—sufficient to prevent the spread of germs.

- Choose nontoxic cleaners. You can find green-friendly cleaners in the grocery store.

- Stop buying pesticides.

A Summary Plan for Minimizing Pesticides in Your Life

- Remove all products from your home designed to kill living things, even bugs, pests, and bacteria, and stop buying them.[125]
- Rely on prevention, cleanliness, and exclusion to prevent pests in the house.[126]
- Eat organic foods. These are raised with pesticides from natural sources.
- Avoid genetically modified organisms (GMOs)—
  a main purpose of GMOs is to allow more effective use of pesticides.
- Choose nontoxic cleaners. You can find green-friendly cleaners in the grocery store.
- Don't use chemicals on your lawn.
- Don't use toxic insect repellants.

To counteract the effects of pesticides encountered elsewhere:

- Take antioxidant supplements like vitamin C, E, CoQ-10, and alpha-lipoic acid.
- Exercise.

Toxins in Personal Care Products

Using personal care products on your face or body is pretty much the same as eating that product. If you doubt me, rub raw garlic on the bottom of your foot. You will soon be tasting it in your mouth.

Before you leave your house in the morning, you may have already faced exposure from harmful chemicals in soaps, shampoo, cosmetics and other personal care products.[127] Many of these have severe consequences for your health and well-being.

Be warned: Many companies that label their products as "organic" or "natural" base this claim on a favorable, self-serving interpretation while hiding many of their ingredients.

For the sake of your brain, take a close look at the ingredients. The following table offers information on harmful chemicals in personal care products.

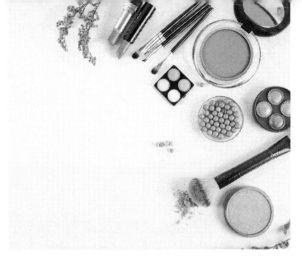

What you put on your face or body can make its way into your body and cause damage. Buy with caution!

TABLE: Harmful Chemicals is Personal Care Products, Where They are Found, Health Effects and How to Avoid Them

Harmful Chemical	Where Found	Health Effects	How to Avoid
1,4-Dioxane	• Shampoos • Body washes • Lotions	• Kidney toxicant • Neurotoxicant • Lung irritant • Carcinogen	• Buy products certified under the USDA National Organic Program.
Parabens	• Deodorants and antiperspirants • Shampoos and conditioners • Spray tans • Lotions and sunscreens • Makeup and other cosmetics • Pharmaceuticals • Food additives • Fragrances	• Endocrine disruptor • Estrogen mimic • Breast cancer risk	• Look for paraben-free products to purchase. • Look for products in dark containers with a pump to keep out light and air. • Use products before their expiration date.
Phthalates (Phthalates make cosmetics easy to spread; now banned in products for children under four years of age. More than 90% of people have detectable levels in their urine.[128])	• Nail polish and removers • Hairsprays • Lipstick • Shampoos • Perfumes	• Mitochondrial damage • Low sperm count • Possible liver damage	• Don't use plastic products with recycling codes of 3 and 7. • Avoid using any plastic in the kitchen. • Use glass, stainless steel, or silicone. • Look in ingredient lists and avoid products containing phthalates.

Harmful Chemical	Where Found	Health Effects	How to Avoid
Methylisothiazolinone (MIT) (Kills bacteria and fungi)	• Shampoos • Conditioners	• At higher concentrations, linked to diseases of the brain and nervous system • Allergen • Irritant	• Look online for MIT-free hair care products.
Toluene	• Synthetic fragrances • Nail polishes	• Neurological damage • Impairs breathing • Causes nausea • Liver and kidney damage • Developmental problems in fetuses • Low blood cell counts	• Check online to verify your favorite products are free of "the toxic three": toluene, dibutyl phthalate and formaldehyde. • Be careful of products applied at a salon, especially if there is inadequate ventilation. • At home, apply nail polish in a well-ventilated room.
Triclosan	• Some dish soaps • Toothpaste • Shampoos • Acne treatments	• Mitochondrial damage • Disrupts hormones • Impaired muscle function • A possible contribution to antibiotic-resistant germs	• Avoid products labeled as "antibacterial." • Check online for Triclosan-free personal care products.
Sodium lauryl sulfate (SLS) and aluminum lauryl sulfate (ALS)	• Shampoos • Laundry detergents • Dish soaps • Toothpaste	• Irritation to eye and skin • Possible allergen	• Check online for SLS and ALS-free personal care products.

Harmful Chemical	Where Found	Health Effects	How to Avoid
Propylene glycol	• Skin conditioning agents • Fragrances • Cosmetic moisturizers • Shampoos	• Possible irritant and allergen	• If you are developing allergies, you may want to find products that are free of this chemical.

Ingredients to Avoid
Organized by Personal Care Product

Protect yourself and your loved ones by checking the following products for ingredients to avoid:

Product	Ingredients to avoid
Bath oils/salts:	lauryl sulfates
Body wash:	1,4-dioxane, Triclosan, lauryl sulfates
Conditioners:	parabens
Cosmetics:	parabens, phthalates, toluene, Triclosan, propylene glycol
Deodorants:	parabens, Triclosan
Detergents:	phthalates, lauryl sulfates
Hair dye:	lauryl sulfates
Lotions:	1,4-dioxane, parabens
Lubricants:	phthalates
Perfume:	phthalates
Shampoo:	1,4-dioxane, parabens, Methylisothiazolinone, lauryl sulfates, propylene glycol
Soaps:	Triclosan, lauryl sulfates
Spray tans:	parabens, toluene
Sunscreens:	parabens
Toothpaste:	Triclosan, lauryl sulfates

A Final Word on Personal Products

What I am describing is a lifetime journey, not only for you, but also for your kids, parents, family, friends and neighbors. The following websites may help. (Editor's note: The author has no financial interest in any of them.)

- SafeCosmetics.org: Personal products
- ewg.org: Food, cleaning products
- Honest.com: Cleaning products

Tobacco—An Addictive Toxin

Tobacco is unmistakably the single most significant cause of preventable death on the planet. We have created many ingenious methods for getting tobacco into our system: chewing and snorting, pipes, cigars, snuff and hookah pipes. The most common of these practices today is smoking cigarettes.

Each cigarette has more than 500 biologically active components, including tar, carbon monoxide, formaldehyde, ammonia, hydrogen cyanide, arsenic and DDT. The smoke alone from cigarettes contains over 4,000 chemicals, many of them causing cancer (which is why second-hand smoke is so dangerous).[129]

Nicotine

When smoked, the nicotine travels from the lung to the brain in about 10 seconds. Nicotine's effects on the brain only last for about 20 to 30 minutes. For those brief moments, what it does makes life seem better for the smoker:

- It serves as a stimulant, making smokers feel more energized—at least for those 20 or 30 minutes.
- Because of specialized receptor cells in the brain, nicotine helps people relax, settle anxieties, feel better and think more clearly—again only for those brief minutes.

These two effects feel good, but nicotine's long-term effect is deadly.

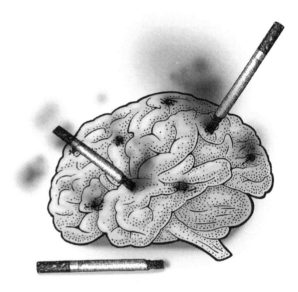

Tobacco is a major risk factor for Alzheimer's because it "rusts" the cells in your brain.

Nicotine Addiction

One reason nicotine is so addictive is because smokers' brains continually develop new receptors in the brain. If smokers don't continually "feed" these receptors, smokers get anxious and irritable until they smoke another cigarette.

Even worse, when smokers are under a lot of stress, a hormone called corticosterone decreases the effects of nicotine. Then smokers need to smoke more and more frequently to get that release from anxiety and discomfort.

Nicotine and Your Brain

Smoking causes oxidative stress in the brain.

To review, oxidation occurs when an invasive atom or molecule steals an electron from another atom. Nicotine is one of the "invaders" who does this. The theft results in a chain reaction of damage as atoms keep stealing electrons from other nearby atoms.

Increased oxidation, or "rusting," is one of the most consistent markers for Alzheimer's dementia.[130]

Smoking also decreases the blood supply to the brain. This limits oxygen and nutrients for neurons and leads to eventual cell death.

I look forward to a time when doctors will regularly assess their patients' risk of Alzheimer's dementia. When doctors do begin doing risk assessments for dementia, I'm sure smoking will be high on the list. If you smoke, your brain begs you to stop!

Nicotine and Your Overall Health

Smoking tobacco causes heart attacks, stroke, COPD, throat cancer, bladder cancer, pancreatic cancer, hypertension, peripheral vascular disease, miscarriages, erectile dysfunction and (indirectly) sudden infant death syndrome and low birth weight for babies.

Eliminate this one risk factor from your life, and your health and well-being will improve dramatically.

Bottom line

For your own sake and for the health of the people you live with, please, if you don't smoke, DON'T START! If you do smoke, QUIT. Your doctor can help.

Medications

As a doctor, I prescribe medications every day, and I am a survivor because of medication. And yet every time I write out a prescription, I have to weigh the medication's benefit against its risks. My default position is to try to find another treatment.

Why? *Because all medications cause some level of damage even as they heal.*

Medications are intentionally designed to interfere with "normal cellular processes." In other words, they are deliberately designed to damage cells that are contributing to a disease.

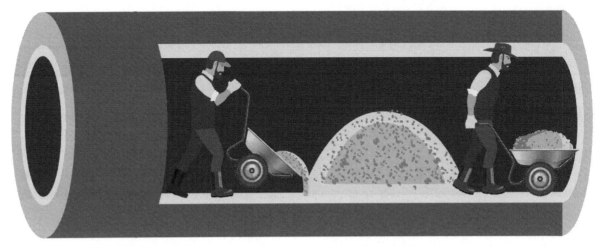

Two transport vehicles: Low-density lipoproteins (LDL) deposit cholesterol in your arteries. High-density lipoproteins (HDL) carry it away.

The medical world has learned to use these harmful substances to our advantage, and sometimes we need them to save our lives. Because of their risks, please be careful. Even the best medications will cause problems if taken incorrectly or needlessly.

With regard to your brain, I am especially concerned about the following medications.

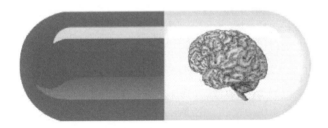

Medications can hold your brain hostage. Be careful to take them as prescribed.

Cholesterol Medications

I'm sorry that cholesterol has such a bad name in our society. It helps to maintain proper hormonal balance in the body, it's a building block for human tissue, and it supports good liver function.

Cholesterol is vital to the brain and especially your memory. In fact, among older people, those with highest cholesterol levels had the best memory function.[131] And yet, millions of people take medication every day to decrease their overall levels of cholesterol. You may be one of them.

Doctors prescribe these medications, called "statins," to decrease levels of bad cholesterol, but by doing so, they limit the cholesterol that your brain so desperately needs. Let me explain.

Cholesterol has two main "transport vehicles"

Cholesterol is produced in the liver. An integral part of cell membranes, it is found in most body tissues. It travels throughout your body via the blood.

Two main kinds of transport vehicles, or lipoproteins, carry the cholesterol through your blood.

1. ***Low-density lipoproteins (LDL):*** We refer to LDL cholesterol as "bad." It leaves thick, hard deposits of cholesterol in your arteries called plaque.

If enough plaque develops, your arteries become clogged. Think of LDL cholesterol as poorly maintained trucks that deposit scummy fluids everywhere they go. The clogged arteries that result from LDL contribute to heart problems and strokes.

2. ***High-density lipoproteins (HDL):*** We consider HDL cholesterol "good." It comes along and removes all the debris LDL leaves in the bloodstream. HDL then takes the debris to the liver where it can be broken down.

The Problem with Statins

Statins are a medication prescribed for patients with elevated cholesterol. Many physicians believe reducing cholesterol lessens the risk of heart disease and stroke. This solution may seem simple, but it is steeped in controversy because statins decrease both good and bad cholesterol.

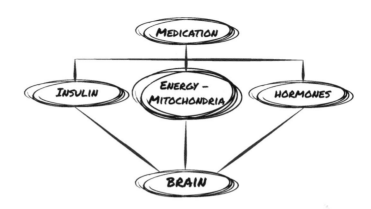

Your medications could be affecting your brain.

The brain has more cholesterol than any other part of your body—almost 25% of your total body cholesterol—so when statins interfere with the production of cholesterol in the liver, problems ensue.

Your brain needs this cholesterol to balance hormone production, improve mitochondrial function, and keep the insulin signaling system operating correctly in the brain.[132]

You can think of cholesterol as the music accompanying the complex dance performance going on in your brain. Cholesterol medication strikes a discordant chord reverberating throughout your body. It:

- Disrupts the healthy metabolism of lipids in the whole body
- Impedes the production and function of healthy hormones
- Decreases optimal insulin function
- Decreases the coenzyme Q10 (CO-Q10), which is an essential element for producing energy in your cells' mitochondria

How to minimize the effects of statins

First, do not go off or decrease your dosage of statins until you speak with your doctor. Your doctor knows your history and is better able to advise you on medications than I am.

When you discuss this with your doctor, you could ask what you can do to address your risk of heart attack and stroke in another way. Here are some suggestions:

- Exercise
- Reduce refined grains and sugars in your diet
- Eat a variety of fruits and vegetables
- Increase fiber
- Limit unhealthy fats
- Cook mindfully
- Maintain a healthy weight

Begin taking Coenzyme Q10 (CO-Q10). This supplement can reduce statin side effects.

Anticholinergics

These include over-the-counter medications including sleep aids like diphenhydramine (the blue tablet often taken to help people get to sleep), motion sickness remedies and allergy medications.

These drugs block a neurotransmitter called acetylcholine in the central and peripheral nervous system. Recent studies have established a strong association between this category of medications and dementia, perhaps related to a decrease in brain size.[133]

The effect on older adults is stronger than it is on younger people. Please seek another treatment!

The Problem with Overmedicating

Doctors want to help their patients, so they generally pay close attention to side effects, prescribing doses designed to halt the disease without doing damage through side effects.

Unfortunately, without realizing it, many older patients have too many overlapping medications, and often at inappropriate dosage levels. If a patient has multiple doctors, or if patients don't disclose all their medications, a doctor might mistakenly prescribe a duplicate or unnecessary medication.

This also happens more often now that pharmaceutical companies can market their medications directly to consumers. We all want quick fixes. It takes a bold doctor to refuse patients seeking a drug and to tell them instead to make lifestyle changes. (If you have one of those doctors, thank him or her during your next office visit.)

You can have a role in avoiding overmedicating.

How to Avoid Overmedicating

- Make a list of all your medications, including over-the-counter medicines, supplements and vitamins. Keep it with you and updated.

- Always take this list when you see a doctor. Once or twice a year, ask your doctor to review it for any potential drug interactions or medications you should stop taking. Many doctors do this without being asked.
- When being prescribed a new medication, discuss side effects and potential interactions with your doctor or pharmacist.
- Set up a tried-and-true system for organizing your medications to be sure you take them on schedule.
- Report problems from medications, including any cognitive results (brain fogginess, memory problems, confusion, etc.). Go to your nearest emergency room if you experience a severe reaction.
- If necessary, you can make an appointment for a "medication check-up" with your pharmacist. Most pharmacies have someone on staff who holds a Doctor of Pharmacy degree (Pharm.D.), granted for completion of doctoral studies specializing in medications.[134]

Illicit Drugs and Alcohol

Excessive use of illicit drugs and alcohol (see the section on alcohol in Chapter 14) can lead to a condition called Substance-Induced Persisting Dementia (SIPD).

Symptoms of SIPD include trouble with memory, personality changes, impaired judgment, struggles with language and other symptoms that mimic Alzheimer's.

Fortunately, you can reverse the damage SIPD does if you stop abusing drugs and alcohol. Of course, it's not easy to stop, but there are treatment programs available.

Traumatic Brain Injury

Trauma, a result of environmental dangers, is an unfortunate event in any form. Trauma from a fall, a violent attack, sexual abuse or a car accident changes your brain and may cause increased inflammation, hormone imbalance and disorders like insomnia, anxiety and depression. All of these can contribute to memory impairment and neurodegenerative disease.

Head injuries in young people may be associated with an increased risk of eventual Alzheimer's disease and other forms of dementia. This is especially true for carriers of the apolipoprotein e4 (APOE-e4) allele. After a trauma, APOE-e4 influences neurodegeneration, and both amyloid beta deposition and tau tangling occur.

How to Avoid Brain Injury

- **Wear a helmet** on a bicycle, motorcycle, scooter, skateboard, snowmobile and other vehicles that could cause head injury in an accident. Wear one as well when playing sports and riding horses.

- **Wear a seat belt** in the car and restrain your children properly.

- **Hold on to the rail** when you go downstairs.

- **Practice gun safety.**

- **Clear pathways and stairs.**

- **Play sports as safely as possible.** Wear a safety helmet when biking, follow the rules at swimming pools and on diving boards and avoid playing American football altogether.

- **Don't drink and drive** or ride in a car driven by someone who's been drinking.

- **As you age, practice your balance.** Here's a simple exercise. (If you feel at all unsteady, have someone nearby to catch you if you begin to fall.) Put your hands on your waist. Lift one leg sideways a couple of inches off the floor, then bring it back down. Repeat ten times on one leg. Then do the other leg. Switch three times for a total of 30 lifts for each leg. Ask your doctor for additional exercises.

- **Avoid standing on a step stool if at all possible.**

- **Install grab bars by your bathtub.** Use non-slip mats as well.

- **Ask your doctor to check your medications** for any prescription drugs that might cause you to fall.

- **Begin an exercise program:** Preferably, start a program that gives you a chance to work on balance—but please, be careful not to fall.

Electromagnetic Fields (EMFs)

This term describes the combined radiation that emanates from electrical appliances, power lines, home wiring, cell phones, radio, TV and Wi-Fi transmitters.

According to some experts, the combined force of all this radiation, both non-ionizing and ionizing, can be damaging to our health. The byproducts of energy-efficient computers, refrigerators and other appliances can be especially harmful.[135]

There's also a high correlation between occupational exposure to electromagnetic fields and dementia.[136] Scientists are studying what might cause this close association.

Perhaps EMFs affect calcium homeostasis. This can activate immune cascades and inflammatory responses that affect neuronal degeneration and dementia. EMFs may also affect insulin receptor sensitivity and aggregating amyloid fibrils.

Others claim the connection occurs because of dental materials in your mouth. Mercury amalgams, metal crowns, dentures and implants may respond to EMFs in a way that contributes to dementia.

Whatever the cause, I suggest you seek to minimize your exposure to electromagnetic fields.

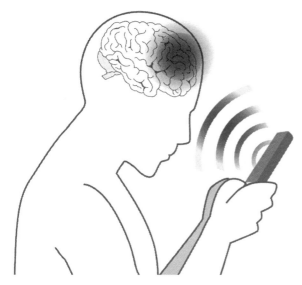

Be mindful of the effects of electromagnetic fields.

How to Avoid or Reduce Exposure to Electromagnetic Fields

CreateYourHealthyHome.com provides many of the following suggestions.[137] If EMF exposure concerns you, this website has a great deal of helpful information, including how to measure EMF levels in your home. (I have no financial interest in this organization.)

- *Try to keep electricity contained in wires:* This means no cordless phones, no wireless technology, no mobile phones, television, radio transmitters or Bluetooth headsets.

- *Avoid using magnets around your body.*

- *Put your laptop on a table rather than your lap.*

- *Use cable instead of wireless technology*: If you do use wireless, turn your router off at night.

- *Use land-line phones—not a cordless phone*: If you must use a mobile phone, use it several inches away from your body.

- *Recharge your devices as far as possible from areas in which you spend the most time*: That means away from your bed, armchair and kitchen.

- *Don't use a microwave oven.*

- *Use only lower-energy halogen bulbs.*

- *Turn off your tablet at night.*

- *Don't ever use dimmer switches.*

- *Unplug appliances when not in use.*

Other Toxins

The following table offers information on many other toxins that you can remove from your life to reduce your risk of Alzheimer's. These tables also list the source and health effects of these toxins, and how to avoid them.

TABLE: Toxins, Their Sources, Health Effects and How to Avoid Them

Toxin	Source	Health Effects	How to Avoid
Aluminum	• Deodorants • Foil wrap • Food additive in beverages, baking powder, processed cheese and pancake/waffle mix • Antacids • Cookware	• Possible link to a higher risk of Alzheimer's • Neurofibrillary degeneration • Possible memory loss	• Use stainless steel cookware, utensils and food containers. • Use deodorants without aluminum. • Get enough calcium to inhibit aluminum absorption. • Filter your water.
Atrazine (especially a hazard to those living in agricultural areas)[138]	• Groundwater	• Neurotoxin • Endocrine disruptor	• Buy organic produce. • Filter your water.
Arsenic (Arsenic occurs naturally in the earth's crust, although usually at low levels.)	• Tobacco • Some commercially raised chickens • Treated lumber • Some cancer treatments	• Neurotoxin • Endocrine disruptor • Damage to all major organs with long-term exposure	• Stop smoking. • Filter your water.
BPA and BPS	• Plastic and canned products (unless marked BPA/BPS-free)	• Toxic to mitochondria • Mimics estrogen	• Avoid plastic and canned products. • Eat fresh food • Use silicone, glass or stainless-steel containers. • Never microwave in plastic containers.

Toxin	Source	Health Effects	How to Avoid
Cadmium (The glaze on some ceramics may contain cadmium.)	• Tobacco • Polluted drinking water • Ni-cadmium batteries if corroded or broken	• Accumulates in the brain • Neurological damage • Inhibits formation of enzymes • Affects action of nutrients	• Stop smoking. • Filter your water. • Keep batteries away from children.
Chlordane	• Left over from pesticide banned in 1983 • Left over from termite control banned in 1988	• Neurological damage	• Avoid digging around older houses where termite control previously included the use of chlordane.
Dioxin (The USDA describes dioxins as "ubiquitous and persistent in the environment.")[139]	• Receipts • Dairy products • Meat and poultry • Eggs • Fish • Animal fats	• Neurological damage • Cancer • Damage to the immune system and hormones • Reproductive problems	• Avoid handling printed receipts from cash registers. • Avoid products high in animal fats.
Flame Retardants	• Children's toys • Baby pillows • Insulation • Foam products • Televisions • Computers	• Damages mitochondria	• Look for products free of retardants. • Get rid of furniture with exposed foam. • Use a HEPA filter to remove dust. • Practice fire safety.

Toxin	Source	Health Effects	How to Avoid
Glycol Ethers	• Paint solvents • Cleaning products • Brake fluid • Cosmetics	• Endocrine disruptors • Lower sperm counts • Allergies and asthma in children	• Be careful with spray products like air fresheners, glass cleaners and other cleaning sprays.
Iron Overload (Usually a result of a genetic disorder)	• Taking too many iron supplements • The inability of the body to process iron correctly • Regular blood transfusions	• Increased risk of infections • Cancer • Arthritis • Heart problems	• Have your iron level monitored by your doctor.
Lead	• Old water pipes • Lead-based paints • Lead storage batteries • Hair dye • Candy from other countries • Lead-glazed pottery • Ammunition • Hobby materials	• Behavioral and learning disorders (ADD, ADHD) • Sensory deficiencies • Motor deficiency • Cognitive dysfunction • Depression • Confusion	• Run water before using. • Filter your water. • Test the paint in your home for lead. • Do not let children play near peeling paint. • Get enough calcium, iron and vitamin C in your diet.

Toxin	Source	Health Effects	How to Avoid
Mercury	• Fish containing mercury • Batteries • Old thermometers and barometers • Certain cosmetics[140] • Some dental fillings[141]	• Fatigue • Moodiness • Anxiety • Depression • Kidney disease • Inflammation of the gut • Memory impairment • Brain atrophy	• Choose wild-caught salmon, pollock, catfish, sardines and anchovies. • Avoid eating fish from the top of the food chain—tuna, shark and king mackerel. • Filter your water. • Request dental fillings without mercury.
PCB (polychlorinated biphenyl) (Banned in 1979)	• Meat, poultry and fish contain residual PCBs.	• Neurological damage	• Avoid animal fat. • Cook fish and meat so the fat can drip away. • Limit dairy fat.
PFCs (perfluorinated chemicals)	• Non-stick cookware	• Endocrine disruption	• Avoid non-stick cookware. • Avoid clothes with water-resistant coatings.
Phthalates	• Plastic storage containers • Garden hoses • Shower curtains • Any plastic tubing	• Mitochondrial damage • Low sperm count • Possible liver damage	• Avoid plastic products with recycling codes of 3 and 7. • Avoid using plastic in the kitchen.

Toxin	Source	Health Effects	How to Avoid
TCE (trichloroethylene)	• Solvents • Production of refrigerants	• Neurological damage • Memory problems • Insomnia • Fatigue	• Avoid spot removers and carpet cleaners.
Toluene (primarily a workplace hazard)	• Paint thinners • Nail polish remover • Glue • Industrial processes	• Neurological damage • Impairs breathing • Causes nausea • Damages the liver and kidney • Produces developmental problems in fetuses • Results in low blood cell counts	• Check online to verify that your favorite products are free of "the toxic three": toluene, dibutyl phthalate, and formaldehyde. • Be careful of products applied at a salon, especially if there is inadequate ventilation. • At home, apply polish in a well-ventilated room.
Triclosan	• Some dish soaps • Toothpaste • Shampoos • Sanitizers • Toys • Acne treatments	• Mitochondrial damage • Disrupts hormones • Impairs muscle function • Possibly contributes to antibiotic-resistant germs	• Avoid products labeled as "antibacterial." • Check online for Triclosan-free personal care products.

Good News about Toxins

This chapter about toxins is long, and threats lurk on every page. I hope you have been able to access information throughout that will help you.

In your efforts to remove toxins from your life, your body provides you with powerful allies in the many different cells and organs that are specialized for removing these toxins from your body.

The liver: This is your body's primary detoxification system. It removes toxic medications, harmful minerals, food additives, toxic byproducts of digestion, foreign invaders like bacteria and viruses and other unwanted products.

But like a soldier who has to challenge too many enemies, your liver can be overwhelmed by too many toxins. Give it a break!

The lymph system and glymphatic system: The lymph system detoxifies your body, and the glymphatic system detoxifies your brain. Both do so at the cellular level. One of the most critical functions of these systems is to defend your body against harmful substances and purify your body and brain fluids.

The kidneys: Your kidneys flush toxins, waste products and harmful chemicals out of your blood. Too many of these harmful waste products can clog up the system and make it hard for your kidneys to do its work. High or low blood pressure also decreases the kidneys'

effectiveness. It's so important to protect your kidneys!

The gut: Besides digestion, the gut's primary purpose is to remove toxins. (See the chapter on the gut, especially its close connection to cognitive health.)

The respiratory tract: Your lungs and bronchi remove toxins that enter your body through your breath.

Your skin: Your skin helps remove toxins in the form of crystals through sweat glands and sometimes through rashes. Exercise that works up a good sweat or even time in a sauna can help cleanse your body of toxins.

Protect Your Allies in the Fight!

All these systems will help you as you seek to detoxify your life and protect your brain, but in return, they need a little help from you:

1. *Decrease your stress*: Stress will limit your liver's ability to detoxify. If you hold on to anger, even a high organic diet will not protect you from toxins. So drop hate. Forgive and love with gratitude.

2. *Detoxify your gut:* First, get the "garbage" out. Eliminate inflammation with nutrient-dense foods that have lots of fiber. A daily bowel movement will cleanse your gut, and when you cleanse your gut, you cleanse your mind.

3. *Give your liver a rest:* The liver is the most ignored

but essential organ in the body. It works nonstop, and nobody pays attention. Stop putting toxins in your body, so it will have a chance to catch up.

4. *For your kidneys, hydrate, hydrate, hydrate:* If water on its own doesn't appeal, try putting in some fresh lemon or lime.

5. *Breathe clean air.:* Your lungs have enough work to do!

6. *Exercise:* This will help clean your lungs, and when you sweat, you'll lose toxins through your skin.

7. *Massage and exercise:* This supports your lymphatic system.

This has been a challenging topic. The world today exposes us to toxins from so many directions. But there is no reason for you to feel helpless. Your body is on your side, and it wants to thrive.

If you maintain your body's detoxifying system, you will find it is precise, efficient and accurate in doing its job.

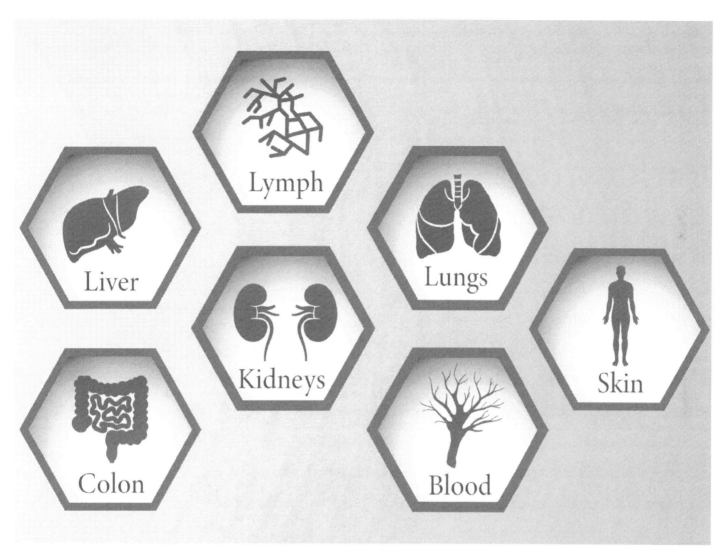

*Seven body organs that work together
to cleanse your body of toxins.*

Chapter 20

Rid Your Body of Hormone Imbalances

Let your hormones dance together and keep your memory sharp.

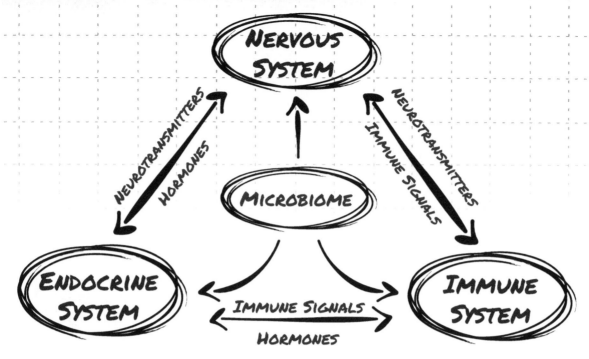

Your hormone system is part of a highly complex communication network.

Your hormones are part of your endocrine system. This highly complex system is affected by many, many variables in your body. In this chapter, I will simplify its role, especially as it relates to dementia. In the end, hormonal balance is what's most important for your brain, memory and overall health.

How Cells Communicate

First, let's review how your cells communicate with each other, with your organs and with the environment around you.

Three major systems are involved in this communication:

1. **The nervous system** uses neurotransmitters to transfer messages to and from your brain and other organs in your body.

2. **The immune system** communicates between groups of immune cells to detect invading or abnormal cells and destroy them.

3. **The endocrine system** uses chemical messengers called hormones to affect the way other cells function.

The interplay of cells within these systems is frequent and well-organized. But if stress or some other disruption affects one of these systems, the others will suffer as well. And then your overall health will suffer.

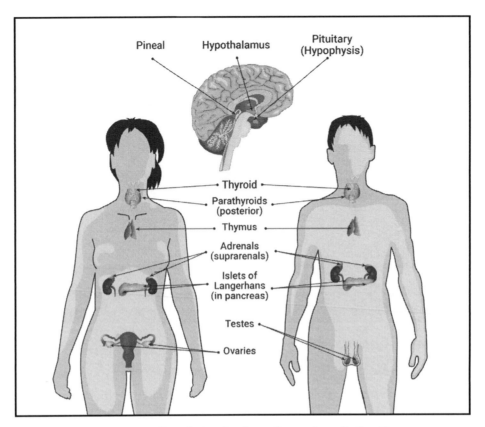

Hormone glands in the female and male bodies

Hormones Working Together

Hormones are chemicals that circulate in your body, regulating your body's function and response to many demands. If you want to be healthy and happy, it's essential that the hormones and chemicals in your body are free to function correctly.

Imagine them as dancers performing highly complicated choreography. When each dancer performs the practiced steps, the dance achieves the desired effect. But when one dancer steps out of place, forgets the routine or loses connection to the music, the entire performance suffers.

That's how it is with your hormones. If everything is in order, in sync, then you have health.

What can disrupt this tightly choreographed dance? Some of the more common disruptions are pictured. I suspect they will look familiar to you!

In this chapter, you will find information and tactics to help you keep your hormones dancing together beautifully.

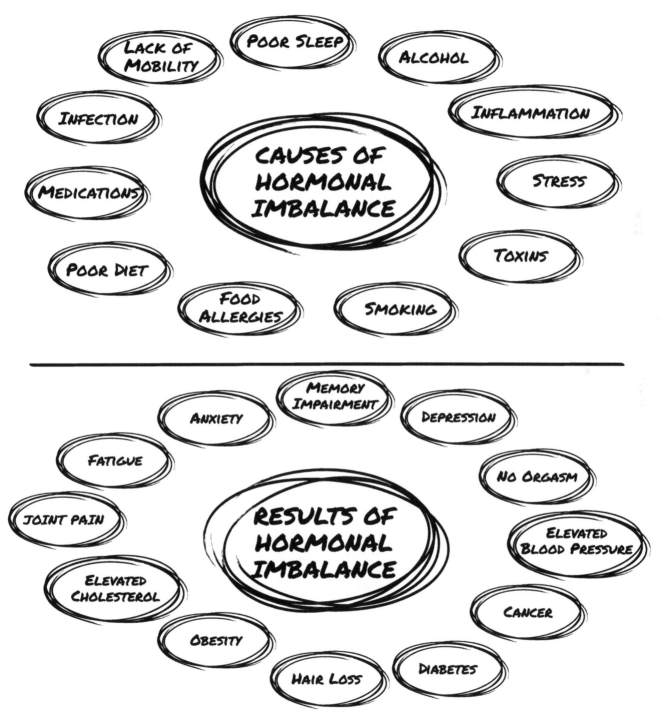

Causes and results are hormonally balanced.

What the Endocrine System Does

The endocrine system controls body processes like growth and development, tissue function, metabolism and sexual function. These glands in your body produce and store hormones: the hypothalamus, thyroid, pancreas, adrenal and pituitary glands in both men and women, and the ovaries in women and testes in men.

When a cell needs to do something, the brain sends a signal to the appropriate gland. This gland releases hormones into the bloodstream. When these hormones reach the correct target cells, the hormones trigger the desired response (or responses).

That is, if everything is working correctly. The problem comes when there's too much or too little of a certain hormone. Each hormone has an optimal range. When hormones fall into that ideal range, your body will receive the best possible benefit.

At other times, a hormone may fail to create the needed response.

Please talk to your doctor!

Your doctor can often discover if hormonal imbalances are present through blood work or other tests. If you do have a hormone imbalance, your doctor may then be able to suggest treatment or help you work on the underlying causes related to your lifestyle.

Sex Hormones

You may think these hormones primarily moderate reproduction, but they do much more. Because oxytocin, for example, increases when you hug your loved ones, it helps you feel more connected and selfless. The net result is decreased inflammation, better-balanced hormones, improved energy and mood and a sharper memory.

So hug your loved ones, close and often!

Sex hormones also improve your enjoyment of sex and enhance your orgasms. This is great for your brain. Good sex is like rebooting your computer. It reduces stress, decreases inflammation and brings your brain in harmony with your environment and body.

Three sex hormones—estrogen, progesterone and testosterone—have a noticeable effect on your brain health. All three hormones are present in both men and women, though to varying degrees.

If you believe your level of any sex hormone is too low or too high, ***talk to your doctor.*** (Ignore all those Internet hawkers selling sex hormone cures on TV!)

Estrogen

Maintaining the proper level of estrogen in your body can reduce your risk of dementia.[142] First, estrogen helps to decrease inflammation in the brain. It also unlocks receptors in the brain and trigger cells to:

- Help regulate the brain's network of signaling pathways
- Improve blood flow and circulation of blood in the brain
- Regulate and transport glucose and sugar in the brain
- Help turn off chronic inflammation from other immune responses

Some studies also indicate that estrogen promotes neuron function and reduces beta-amyloid plaques and other Alzheimer's markers in the brain.

Progesterone

Think of progesterone as the "healing hormone." It is so crucial to optimal brain function that the cells in your brain produce their own supply. Progesterone can:

- Promote repair after injury
- Repair and regenerate the myelin sheath that protects nerve fibers—the very fibers that break down in Alzheimer's dementia
- Limit tissue damage after traumatic brain injury
- Protect and repair the blood-brain barrier

Testosterone

Testosterone is essential to the brain. If you have low levels, an increase in testosterone can improve focus, memory and spatial reasoning in both men and women, even in Alzheimer's patients.

But be warned. If you have normal levels of testosterone, extra testosterone probably won't improve your brain function and may actually harm it.[143]

More than that, you do not want the side effects that come with too much testosterone, including a higher risk of prostate cancer in men, as well as strokes and heart attacks.

Once again, please **speak with your doctor** about whether your levels are low, and pay close attention when your doctor discusses risks and benefits.

Hormones from the Thyroid Gland

Many years ago, miners took a canary with them underground. The canary's distress warned the miners that the carbon dioxide levels were increasing and that they should leave the mines immediately.

*Your thyroid is like a miner's canary—
it warns of developing health problems.*

The thyroid gland is your body's canary because the thyroid can sense danger in your body. Checking thyroid levels at the doctor's office should be as routine as checking your blood pressure. It will help detect hidden infections, inflammation in your body and the presence of autoimmune diseases.

When the thyroid begins to deteriorate, you may have other health problems as well. Someday thyroid function will be the fifth vital sign along with body temperature, pulse rate, respiration rate and blood pressure.

Because there is such a significant overlap between thyroid function and brain function, checking your thyroid levels will be especially helpful if you want to reduce your risk of dementia.

Causes of thyroid problems

- Poor nutrition
- Chronic stress
- Food allergies
- Infections
- Environmental toxins
- A lack of iodine in the diet (addressed in the United States most frequently through iodized salt)
- Loss of part or all of the thyroid through surgery

Thyroid imbalance

Typically, people with *underactive* thyroids experience fatigue, lack of energy, intolerance to cold, dry skin, weight gain, a low heart rate, menstrual irregularity and depression.

People with an overactive thyroid experience sudden weight loss, a rapid or irregular heartbeat, sweating, anxiety and irritability.

Both an underactive and overactive thyroid can affect your memory and ability to think clearly. With a troubled thyroid, thought processes can slow, we might become more forgetful and depression can result—all problems related to the brain.

Treatment for thyroid problems

Good news! Thyroid problems can often be reversed and treated, either by medication or a lifestyle change. The sooner you recognize a problem and get help, the better.

Cortisol Overload

Cortisol is a critical player in the body's response to danger. A release of cortisol energizes you to act quickly and decisively, whether that means fighting or fleeing from a threat. Once you are out of danger, the cortisol should return to normal levels.

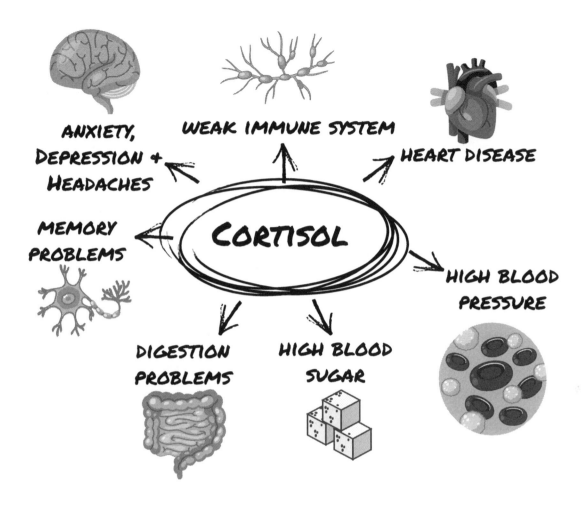

Cortisol overload contributes to a cascade of health problems.

But as you know, our bodies do not always return to normal levels of calm after threats. Instead, anxiety lingers, contributing to chronic inflammation. In these times of continuing, free-floating anxiety, the stress caused by cortisol is an enemy within your gates, causing havoc throughout your body, including your brain.

No wonder people call cortisol the "stress hormone."

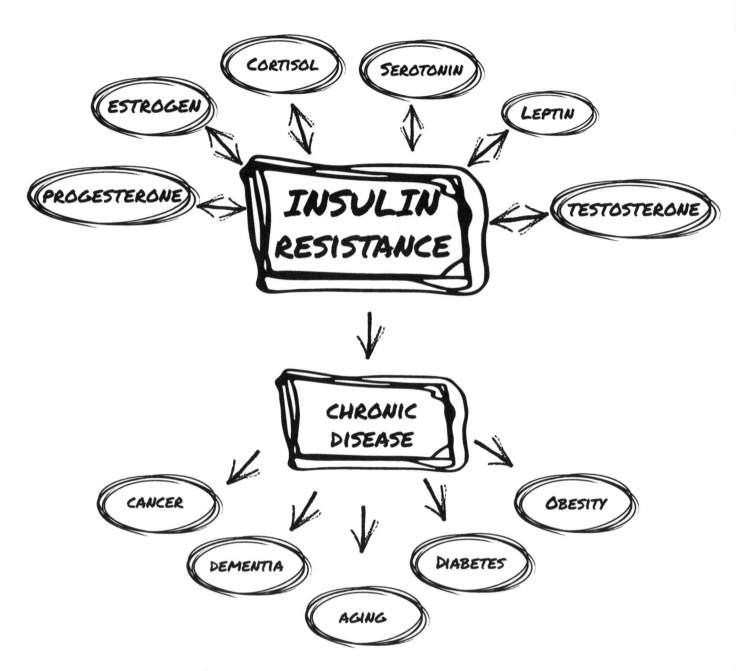

Insulin resistance disrupts many of your hormones and contributes to numerous chronic diseases.

In a healthy body, cortisol levels peak in the morning, telling your body it's time to get up and get moving. They reach their lowest levels in the hours when you sleep.

Predictably, if cortisol stays elevated into the evening, both getting to sleep and staying asleep is more difficult. You probably know from experience how much lack of sleep can interfere with your ability to think. Long-term sleep problems can create long-term problems for your brain, including cell damage and impaired memory retrieval.

In times of chronic stress, your body has to produce extra cortisol, so it shuts down the production of other hormones, creating a significant hormonal imbalance.

It's as if cortisol steals your body's entire hormone budget. The deficits elsewhere result in fatigue and brain fog, memory impairment and many other problems.

Getting your cortisol levels under control is vital for your cognitive health. See the chapter on stress for suggestions.

The All-Encompassing Importance of Insulin and Its Signaling System

Insulin is another hormone that plays a crucial role in your cognitive health. You read about insulin in Chapter 9.

Now that you have learned so much about what increases your risk of Alzheimer's dementia, I want to circle back to sugar, insulin and the insulin signaling system.

A defective insulin-signaling system dramatically increases your risk of Alzheimer's dementia. I hope to convince you to address this risk with all haste.

To review, your body runs on sugar—more specifically, a form of sugar called glucose. The carbohydrates you eat get broken down into glucose so that your stomach and small intestines are able to absorb the glucose. From your stomach and small intestines, the glucose goes into your bloodstream.

But even then our bodies cannot use this glucose. We need insulin to do that. Insulin enters the bloodstream and, like a magic key, a healthy insulin-signaling system unlocks cells and lets sugar in so the cells can use the sugar.

And what if your cells don't need any glucose? Insulin takes care of that as well, by moving the extra glucose into the muscle and liver for storage.

So when everything is working correctly, insulin maintains a steady level of sugar in your blood either by moving it into cells or into the muscle and liver.

Your Insulin Signaling System

This all sounds fairly simple, but the system insulin uses to signal cells to open or to move the sugar into the liver is incredibly complex, involving a cascade of cellular processes—think Niagara Falls, not a gentle trickle.

Unfortunately, under certain circumstances, your body might not produce enough insulin to handle the sugar load in your blood. Or it might resist insulin's attempts to move sugar out of the bloodstream. In both these cases, the insulin-signaling system isn't working properly.

The consequences for our brains are deadly.

Our brain is only 2% of our body, and yet it uses 20% of our energy. It's an energy-guzzling Lamborghini. When your insulin signaling system stops working, the cells can't get the energy they need—sugar, sugar everywhere and none for cells to use.

You probably know what that means. When the insulin-signaling system in the brain isn't working, neurons can't get energy. When neurons can't get enough energy, they die. And when cells die in the brain, you have cleared a path for Alzheimer's dementia.

That's why I believe that improving your insulin signaling system is one of the most urgent and important parts your Dementia Action Plan.

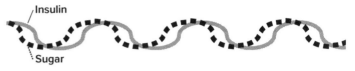

An excellent interplay of sugar (gray) and insulin (black) in the bloodstream. This steady relationship is "the melody of health."

How Our Insulin Signaling System Becomes Damaged

What you really want for your insulin is a nice, steady hum of sugar entering your bloodstream and exiting either to cells or to be stored in the liver—with no sugar spikes and no need for insulin to overreact.

This steady hum of sugar in and out of your bloodstream is the melody of health.

With a diet high in added sugar, processed and fast foods, and unhealthy fats, however, sugar floods into your blood, causing a Def-Con 5 response of insulin.

Sugar goes way, way up, and insulin has to go way, way up as well.

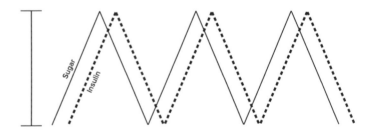

These sudden rises and falls of first sugar and then insulin is the jarring noise of microtrauma.

The net result of these sharp and sudden up-and-down levels of sugar and insulin is a defective insulin signaling system.

Eventually, the body becomes resistant to insulin's efforts to regulate blood sugar. When this happens, you receive a diagnosis of prediabetes or type 2 diabetes.

This diagnosis will increase your risk of Alzheimer's dementia by 50%.

Type 2 diabetes is at an all-time high in the United States. Among people over 65, one out of four people or 25% have type 2 diabetes.

Whether you have been diagnosed with type 2 diabetes or not, this is the time to do everything you can to improve your insulin-signaling system.

Act Now to Improve Your Insulin-Signaling System

In your life, you have things you can change. For health, these *modifiable lifestyle factors* include:

- Improving sleep
- Exercising more
- Eating healthy food
- Decreasing stress
- Breathing clean air, drinking clean water and detoxifying your environment
- Improving relationships
- Increasing sensory and mental stimulation

These are the modifiable lifestyle changes that are available to you for improving a defective insulin signaling system.

Good news! When you address these modifiable lifestyle factors, you will indirectly improve your gut, mitochondria, hormones, immune system/ inflammation, heart and lymph systems and your muscles and bones.

When it comes to your insulin-signaling system, each of these tools separately is powerful, but taken together they will fine-tune your ability to use and store sugar so that your body will sing.

Let's consider each in turn.

Sleep

When you don't get enough good sleep, your body reacts by releasing epinephrine, norepinephrine and cortisol. These hormones cause blood sugar to rise, leading eventually to a defective insulin signaling system. In a particularly vicious cycle, these hormones make it harder for you to get good sleep, and it all happens again.

For the sake of your insulin signaling system, take steps to improve your sleep.

Exercise

Exercise has many advantages for your health. One of the main ones is improving your insulin sensitivity. This makes your cells more willing to respond to the insulin signaling system.

Exercise can also allow your muscles to use sugar more readily. In both cases, this helps regulate the amount of sugar in your blood.

Healthy food

If your blood sugar is consistently high, you can help your insulin-signaling system by avoiding foods that cause a sudden rush of sugar into the blood. This means added sugar, processed food and the four white demons (white rice, white bread, white potatoes and white pasta).

Your body still needs the sugar found in carbohydrates, but if you can eat carbohydrates that combine sugar with fiber, such as fruits, your insulin-signaling system will work better.

Stress

Stress causes the release of these same three hormones that harm your sleep. Decrease your stress to help your insulin signaling system. The chapter on stress gives you many ideas on how to deal with your stress.

Clean air, water and environment

Drinking water and breathing air that is free of toxins and avoiding environmental contaminants will help your insulin-signaling system. The body sees these toxins as dangerous and sends in the troops (inflammatory processes) to try to deal with them.

The result for your blood sugar is simple. Inflamed cells are more likely to resist insulin's attempts to "unlock" the cells. As a result, the insulin-signaling system is thwarted, and the cells can't get the energy they need.

The chapter on toxins offers many suggestions for improving your water, air and environment.

Relationships

I have to admit this has a secondary rather than primary effect on your insulin-signaling system, but I still believe it is very important.

Healthy relationships can bring laughter, joy, comfort, purpose, encouragement and peace into your life. All these offer a respite from the relentless stressors of modern life.

Your social relationships can also provide a powerful motivation for looking after your health, especially if you already have diabetes.

Sensory and mental stimulation

Your thoughts travel on neural pathways through your mind. Sensory stimulation involving your five senses and mental stimulation that involves learning will strengthen and multiply these neural pathways. This will give your thoughts many options for pathways through your brain.

Because this stimulation helps to keep your neurons alive and functioning, it should be part of any dementia action plan, even one focusing on the insulin-signaling system.

From the Roots, the Fruit

These modifiable lifestyle factors are like the roots of a tree that produces your health and well-being. I have shown how dealing with these seven factors can together rejuvenate your insulin-signaling system.

These lifestyle factors can also improve many other chronic diseases if you modify them effectively.

Most of all, making healthy lifestyle changes will dramatically reduce your risk of Alzheimer's dementia. The time to start is now!

Chapter 21

Rid Your Body of Endocrine Disruptors

One out-of-sync dancer disrupts the choreography.

Endocrine-disrupting chemicals (EDCs) interfere with your finely tuned hormones. Some typical examples are BPA and phthalates found in food containers, children's bottles, personal care products and flame retardants.[144]

EDCs fool your body by mimicking hormones and twisting the instructions that the real hormones would have given. They can cause early cell death, compete with essential nutrients and turn one hormone against another.

Some of the most frightening disruptors cause congenital disabilities, but endocrine disruptors can also cause heart disease and many kinds of cancer. Because there's evidence that they also disrupt learning and memory, many experts believe they raise your risk of dementia.

Why are manufacturers allowed to use these dangerous chemicals?

When trying to assess risk, regulatory agencies use the idea that "the dose makes the poison." In other words, if the harmful chemical is present in low enough doses, it's not dangerous.

But how can a safe threshold be established for everyone when our bodies respond so differently and our exposure varies so much?

I never drink water from plastic bottles, for example, but I know people who drink water almost exclusively from them. Doesn't it make sense that what is "generally regarded as safe" for me will be different than what is safe for them?[145]

The American Chemical Society, who knows better than most groups about chemicals and how to test for them, recommends updated testing standards and protocols. The ACS also recommends safer alternatives to endocrine-disrupting chemicals.

For a long time, we thought of these endocrine disruptions as anomalies—strange things that happened without a clear explanation. We now realize that many of these disruptions are environmental, the result of our own choices.

If that's true, you can take steps to avoid them.

To reduce your risk for dementia—and avoid a host of other problems—your best option is to get endocrine disruptors out of your life and the lives of your loved ones.

Doing this won't be easy because they are everywhere—at home, at work, where you shop or dine and where you go to have fun. But small steps in the right direction add up to big changes.

The table below lists several typical endocrine disruptors. I realize it's similar to the table of toxins in the toxins chapter. These toxins, however, are especially threatening to your endocrine system.

TABLE: Endocrine Disruptors, Health Effects and How to Avoid Them

Endocrine Disruptor	Health Effect	How to Avoid
Arsenic	• Interferes with hormone activity in the glucocorticoid system • Can lead to insulin resistance • Can contribute to high blood pressure	• Stop smoking. • Filter your water.
Atrazine	• Linked to breast tumors, delayed puberty • Causes prostate inflammation in animals	• Buy organic produce. • Filter your water.
BPA	• Mimics estrogen • Linked to breast cancer, reproductive problems, early puberty	• Use fresh foods as much as possible. • Avoid canned goods—many food manufacturers line their cans with BPA. • Wash your hands after handling receipts. • Avoid plastics with a recycling code of 7. • Avoid the consumption of contaminated food or water.

Endocrine Disruptor	Health Effect	How to Avoid
Dioxins	• Can affect sperm quality • Can lower sperm count	• Eat fewer animal products. • Avoid handling receipts from cash registers.
Fire Retardants	• Can imitate thyroid hormones	• Look for products free of retardants. • Get rid of furniture with exposed foam. • Use a HEPA filter to remove dust.
Glycol Ethers	• Lower sperm counts • Exposure may result in blood abnormalities	• Wear a mask if you must work with paints or cleaning products that contain glycol ethers. • Check online for cosmetics that do not contain glycol ethers.
Lead	• Linked to premature births and miscarriages • Can disrupt the hormone signaling of the body's primary stress system	• Run water before using. • Filter your water. • Have the paint in your home tested for lead. • Do not let children play near peeling paint. • Get enough calcium, iron and vitamin C in your diet.

Endocrine Disruptor	Health Effect	How to Avoid
Mercury	• Concentrates in the fetal brain • Will bind to hormones involved in menstrual cycles	• Choose wild-caught salmon, pollock, trout, sardines and anchovies. • Avoid fish at the top of the food chain—tuna, shark, swordfish and king mackerel. • Filter your water. • Request dental fillings without mercury.
Organophosphate Pesticides	• Lower testosterone levels • Change thyroid hormone levels • Affect fertility	• Buy organic produce. • Check online for guides to fruits and vegetables with low pesticide residue.
Perfluorinated Chemicals	Linked to the following: • Decreased sperm quality • Low birth weight • Thyroid disease	• Avoid non-stick cookware. • Avoid clothes with water-resistant coatings.

Endocrine Disruptor	Health Effect	How to Avoid
Pesticides (DDT, persistent in the environment, chlorpyrifos, vinclozolin, pyrethroids)	• Mimic natural hormones, causing chemical reactions • Block hormone receptors in cells so that actual hormones cannot function • Affect the synthesis and transport of hormones	• Buy organic produce. • Filter your water.
Phthalates	Linked to the following: • Premature death of testicular cells • Lower sperm count and less mobile sperm • Possibly involved in thyroid irregularities	• Avoid plastic products with recycling codes of 3 and 7. • Avoid using plastic in the kitchen. • Check online for personal care products that don't contain phthalates.
Triclosan	• Disturbs estrogen, testosterone, and thyroid synthesis and distribution • Possible link to early puberty, poor sperm quality and infertility	• Avoid products labeled as "antibacterial." • Check online for Triclosan-free personal care products.

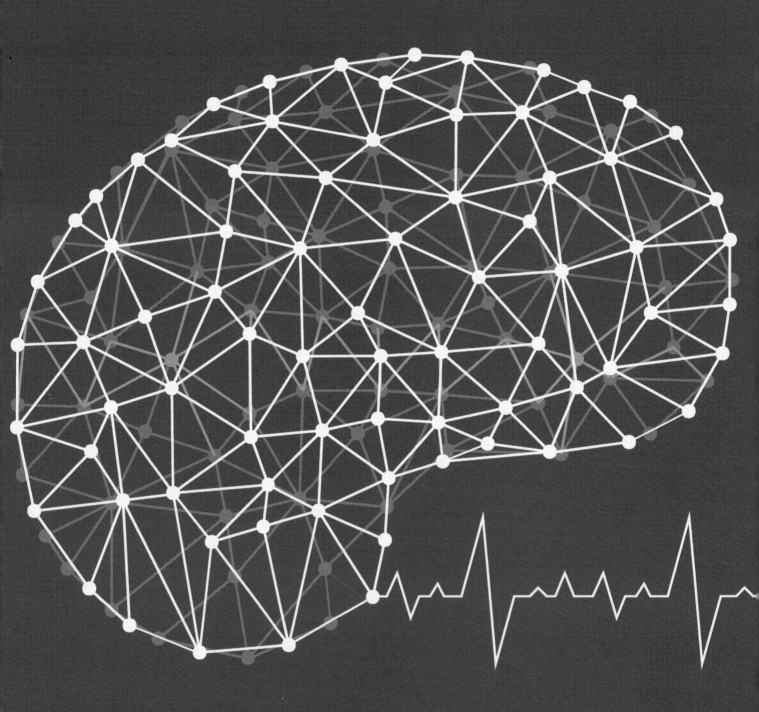

Section 3

Stimulate Your Brain

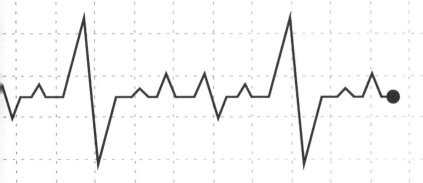

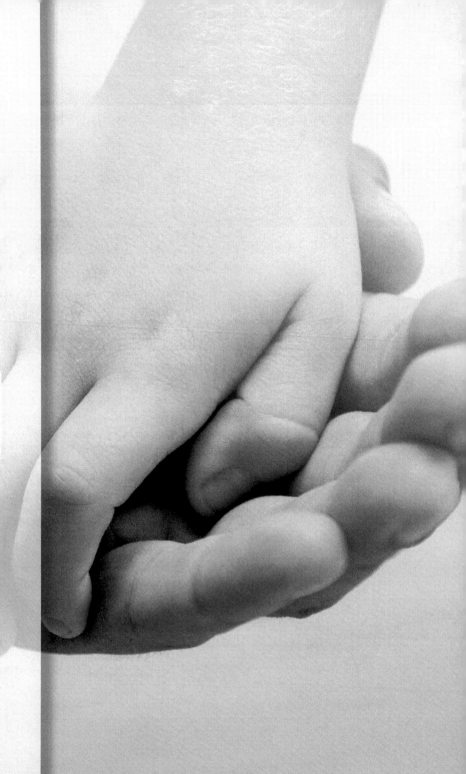

Chapter 22

Social Connection

Let's hold hands.

In my 30s, I came by myself as an immigrant to the United States.

Back in Iran, I had been a practicing physician with friends, family and community connections. In the States, with limited English and cultural barriers all around me, I felt isolated and alone.

In those pre-Skype days, talking to friends and family overseas meant an expensive phone call with no face-to-face contact.

All of that changed one day at the YMCA. An acquaintance saw me, invited me to a music festival, and a new network of friends began for me. As you can imagine, my life became much happier.

Perhaps you have never experienced the abrupt and total isolation I experienced when I came to the States. Maybe your isolation developed gradually— a friend moved away, your children became busy with their own lives or you declined offers for lunch with colleagues too many times, and now they have stopped asking.

If so, your increasing isolation and loneliness will undoubtedly affect your cognitive ability. **Dementia is a social disease and needs a social solution.**

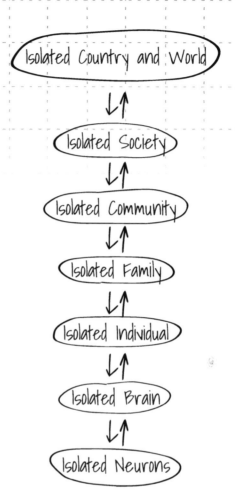

The isolation caused by Alzheimer's affects us from cellular to global levels.

More than just personal happiness and mental comfort, regular social interaction also keeps your brain healthy by triggering numerous neural connections in your brain, keeping the brain nimble.

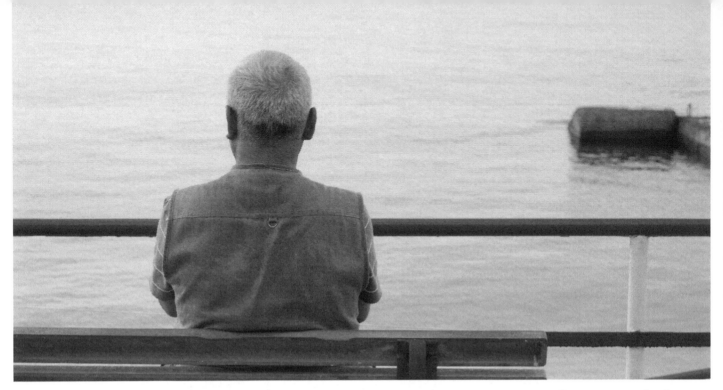

Social connections are so important that daily contact with friends and family can cut your risk of cognitive decline in half.[146]

At this point, please allow me to veer a little into the metaphysical. The beta-amyloid plaques that are so characteristic of Alzheimer's dementia isolate neurons from each other. As the plaques multiply, they eventually isolate a person from his or her memories, and then from this person's loved ones, community and world.

This is the heartache of Alzheimer's dementia. But please notice from the chart on the previous page that the process can go both ways.

Alzheimer's results in isolation. The opposite is also true. Isolation can result in Alzheimer's.

Social connections are vitally important for the health of your brain. Take steps today to avoid isolation and loneliness.

Social Relationships and Your Brain

We don't know exactly how social interactions ward off Alzheimer's, but the theory is that interacting with friends stimulates our thinking in many useful ways.

Even a basic conversation with friends and family requires quick decisions, appropriate choices of words and nonverbal responses. More complex interactions affect your emotions, exercising your ability to respond appropriately with laughter, sorrow, surprise, empathy or curiosity. All of these responses require memory, attention and self-control.

In this way, social interactions exercise your brain and help to create new nerve cells. Healthy social interactions can also stave off depression, anxiety and stress, all of which are associated with cognitive decline.

A word for the introverts among us

If you are an introvert, this advice to have a more active social life may concern you. But I'm not suggesting that you try to remake yourself into an extrovert.

Extroverts gain energy from other people and love being around them, so they usually have a large circle of friends and many social engagements. Introverts, on the other hand, gain energy from solitude and prefer a smaller circle of friends.

Are you under the impression that it's the number of your social contacts that will determine your risk of Alzheimer's? Don't believe it. It's not the size of your social circle that matters but *the quality of your social interactions.*

Some introverts feel most comfortable interacting almost exclusively with their family and a few friends. If that's true for you, that's fine. Interact often, share your life with them, enjoy long conversations and laugh often.

Your interaction with them will help keep Alzheimer's at bay. Grandchildren are especially good at keeping your brain agile.

If you try instead to become an extrovert, you may actually increase your risk of Alzheimer's dementia. Pushing yourself this way will wear you out emotionally, increase your stress and may even depress you.

Introverts who overload on social interactions report brain fog as the evening progresses—the last thing your brain needs. Some even speak of an "introvert hangover."[147]

The world needs introverts, so cherish yourself and your healthy relationships.

How to Limit Isolation's Harmful Consequences

Developing new relationships after the death of a spouse, starting a new job or moving to a new location is hard, but it's possible, and it will do so much good for your cognitive health.

Here are a few suggestions:

How to expand your circle of friends

- *Get involved.* Join a book club at the library, a knitting group, a cooking class, a creative gym for crafting, a synagogue, mosque or church— anywhere that you might find people who share your interests. Once there, open up to people, take part in social opportunities, say "Yes," when someone asks you to join them for a meal. Better yet, initiate social contact. You would be amazed to know how many people are hoping for an invitation.

- **Volunteer.** There's nothing like working for a common cause to build social ties.

How to strengthen your relationships with family and friends

Schedule interactions: Life gets busy. Texting a friend or scheduling a time to call ensures you'll sustain a relationship.

Nurture relationships with friends and family: A sudden frost can kill fragile plants, so gardeners take steps to protect them. Friendships are also "fragile," and we often forget that hurt feelings, blunt comments and a host of other personal failings can damage close relationships.

Protect your relationships by deciding beforehand that you will overlook weaknesses, forgive shortcomings and be quick to reach out again if someone has hurt your feelings—or if you've done the hurting.

Expect less: It is very painful if we do something for friends or family members, and they respond with less appreciation than we wanted—if at all. They don't call on our birthdays. They fail to show up to parties. They don't reply to an invitation.

Friends make mistakes, and sometimes you have to find your pleasure in the generosity you bestow rather than what you get from friends.

Remember: Throughout your friendships, you may have made some mistakes as well.

Forgive: The closer the bond, the more essential forgiveness becomes. That's because eventually all friends or family members hurt each other.

When you are the wounded one, it's helpful to remember, first, that you've done your share of wounding.

It's also worthwhile to remember that forgiving is a choice you make for yourself as much as for your friend. When you forgive, you set aside the heavy burden of carrying a grudge. You also let go of the toxic fury that can control your thoughts and rob you of happiness.

Forgiveness, even if your friend doesn't apologize, can improve your health, decrease your stress, lower your blood pressure, improve your sleep and strengthen your immune system.[148]

A Final Note About Technology

As I have grown older, I have seen more and more disadvantages to technology. Social media, for example, may increase our contacts with each other, but not our deep connections.

If we're not careful, technology can divide and isolate us. The next time you're in a restaurant, notice how many people are looking at their cell phones rather than talking to each other. Yes, we communicate with each other, but only if we can say it quickly in a text.

Technology isn't the problem. It's the way we use it. If used correctly, technology can help decrease our isolation.

Skype, for example, can be an excellent way for family members who live apart to speak face to face.

When my friend's daughter was in China for a year, the family opened Christmas presents on Skype and even watched movies together with a computer set up in front of the television.

This same friend often does the *New York Times* crossword puzzle together with another daughter and reads books to her grandchildren who live three states away.

I encourage you to be intentional with your use of technology so that its effect on your life is enhanced, and so that it diminishes, rather than increases, your risk of Alzheimer's.

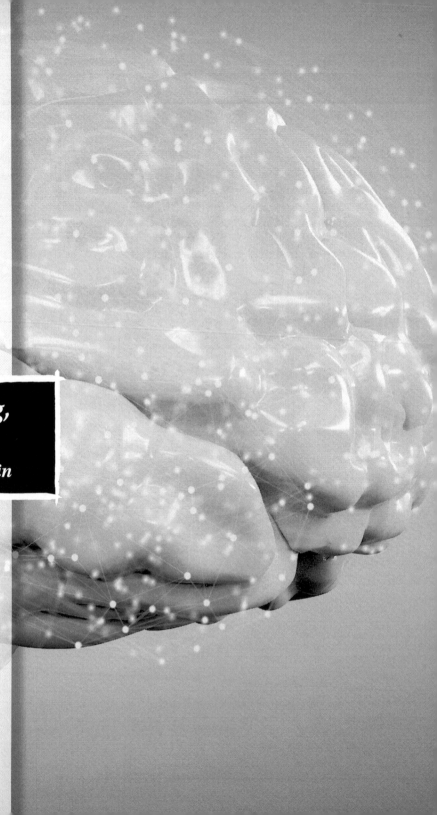

Chapter 23

Keep
Learning

> *"Once you stop learning,*
> *you start dying."*
> **- Albert Einstein**

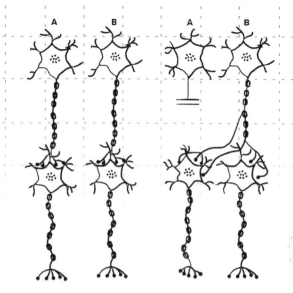

With plenty of available neural pathways, your brain can sidestep any disruption caused by plaques or tangles.

In 1986, David Snowden began a long-term study of 678 nuns, funded by the National Institute on Aging. He did regular tests on physical and cognitive health, and when the nuns died, they donated their brains for further study by autopsy.

Something surprising showed up in these autopsies. Although some of the nuns had brains full of amyloid plaques and tau tangles—two of the hallmark characteristics of Alzheimer's dementia—the nuns had shown no signs of Alzheimer's while they were alive.[149]

Neuroscientists believe this is because the nuns had so much *cognitive reserve*. As part of their normal lives, they had many reasons to keep learning. This learning kept many neural pathways active in their brain.

This means if plaques and tangles cut off one neural pathway, they had others available to use for memory, reasoning and continued learning.

It's All About *Neuroplasticity*

This demonstrates their brains' *neuroplasticity*—in other words, their brains' ability to change the way it does things. Based on what we experience, learn or need, the brain can change its structure and organization.

It's a little like physical exercise, but in the brain it isn't muscle that gets stronger. It's the neural pathways.

To use another picture, it's like creating a path through the woods. The more you walk on the path, the easier it is to see the path and to use it to get somewhere.

Because of their continued learning, the nuns had created so many pathways through their brain that when one was blocked, their thoughts simply stepped sideways onto another neural pathway.

This is the explanation neuroscientists offer for the nuns' cognitive health. This neuroplasticity kept the symptoms of Alzheimer's dementia from showing.[150]

Learning Stimulates New Neural Pathways

Learning is like a mental bank account. The more neural pathways you develop and strengthen, the greater your chance of escaping the symptoms of Alzheimer's.

The more you challenge your brain to keep learning, the more your neurons will be able to redirect their messages when a synapse fails.

The density of synapses decreases in patients with cognitive decline, so if this mental activity can help you produce new synaptic connections in your brain, it's a meaningful way to protect your cognitive health.[151]

In fact, according to some experts, people with high mental activity have a 46% lower risk of developing cognitive decline.[152] You can join them, but you do need the right kind of learning for this to succeed.

Learning Stimulates New Growth

Mental activity is anything that stimulates your brain. It can be provided internally by thinking about something or externally from your environment.

Your social contacts, work, leisure and educational activities can all contribute to your mental activity. So does meditation.

Dr. Lara Lazar, a Harvard neuroscientist, studied the effects of meditation on 16 volunteers. After eight weeks of meditation, brain scans showed that the part of the brain associated with learning and memory had denser gray matter.

Dr. Lazar concluded, "If you use a particular part of your brain, it's going to grow because you are using it. What we are talking about is a form of mental exercise. The idea is 'use it or lose it.' It's like building a muscle."[153]

Another study compared London taxi drivers and bus drivers. To get their taxi permits, taxi drivers have to memorize a map of London with 25,000 streets and thousands of landmarks and then pass a test. The test is so hard that it can take up to 12 attempts to pass it.

In the process of this learning, the taxi drivers gained gray matter in the brains, increased their ability to remember, and added many more neurons to their brains' hippocampus.[154]

As they continued to put this vast learning into use, according to the study, taxi drivers' gray matter continued to increase.

Bus drivers, on the other hand, navigate a fixed route through London and rarely need to learn anything new for their career. In the study, they were shown to have significantly less gray matter.[155]

"Less gray matter" indicates a smaller brain, another hallmark of Alzheimer's dementia.

Two Effects of Learning on Your Brain

Studies like these (there have been others) have caused scientists to conclude that continued learning:

1. Builds new neural networks in your brain

2. Increases gray matter in the brain, which means less shrinkage

The Learning That Protects Your Brain

If you want to protect your brain from the damage of Alzheimer's, learning is essential—but not just any kind of learning. To effectively protect your brain, learning needs four characteristics.

1. Learning has to be new.

As you work toward mastering a new skill, such as learning the Norwegian language or processing information like the history of World War II, the parts of your brain involved with learning and memory expand.

Scientists can measure this expansion with brain scans.

For those of us seeking to avoid Alzheimer's, this is terrific news. Neuroscientist Jason Castro addressed learning and memory expansion when he said, "Practice makes bigger, and bigger means better."[156]

There's a twist, however.

Once you master a skill or content area, your brain stops growing. If you don't keep learning something new, your brain actually retracts to its normal size. And remember, as you age, "normal" means smaller and smaller.

If atrophy and smaller brain size typically come with age, maintaining the growth that you gained from the mental activity is extremely important. You can only do this by learning new skills or knowledge.

Imagine you have been learning to play the piano. In time, you are able to play a fairly challenging piece of music—perhaps "Moonlight Sonata" by Beethoven or perhaps "Jailhouse Rock," if that's more to your taste.

You can now sit down and play the piece *almost without thinking*. If you barely need to think, do you see how the neural pathways necessary to play that piece of music have been established and that you are no longer learning?

In response, your brain retracts to its normal size.

To keep your brain strong, you need to continually push your brain to create new neural pathways. You can do this by moving on to another difficult song and then another one.

You may even want to learn something completely new.

2. Learning has to have an element of difficulty.

Neuroscientist Lisa Feldman Barrett studies "super agers"—people in their 60s and 70s whose brains are as sharp as 25-year-olds.[158]

For one research project, her team used functional magnetic resonance imaging (fMRI) to study the brains of people in this group. She wanted to know why these super agers did not show the typical brain atrophy or thinning that comes with age.

Her conclusions? Vigorous physical exercise combined with strenuous mental effort kept super agers' brains young.

So if you want to be more like the super agers, work your body hard—until you are breathless and "feel the burn." And then work your mind just as hard.

Working your mind means picking something to learn that won't come quickly and is more than just diverting, like puzzles or computer games (more on that later).

Take an astronomy class at the community college (or Shakespeare if you tend naturally to the arts). Memorize poetry, scripture or even your grocery list. Master chess.

Most of all, step out of your comfort zone, and if it's temporarily unpleasant and challenging—fantastic! That's exactly what your brain needs.

"Do it till it hurts," Barrett says, "and then a bit more."[157]

3. Learning should involve more than one sense.

If you involve only sight in your learning, that's one level of difficulty. If you add smell, hearing, taste and touch, it becomes a multisensory experience—and that is so much better.

Multisensory learning requires the brain to reorganize itself and make new connections throughout the brain. ***This is precisely what you want for your cognitive health*** because your brain has been designed to involve all your senses.

Learning a new cooking technique can be multisensory. Consider pastry. You mix the butter, flour, salt and water using your arms. With your eyes, you see if the mixture resembles breadcrumbs. With your hands, you form the mixture into a ball. You follow directions to chill and then roll out the dough. Eventually, you taste the cooked pastry and feel the flakiness in your mouth.

Cooking offers many opportunities for multisensory learning. Woodworking, auto mechanics, knitting and playing the piano do as well. The opportunities for multisensory learning are almost unlimited.

And if you add some friends or acquaintances to this learning, all the better!

4. Learning should include your imagination

As children, you were probably told to stop imagining things. Not anymore.

Imagination allows us to see pictures, create stories, manipulate ideas, make plans and transport ourselves to a world that exists only in our minds. This magical process has remarkable effects on your brain.

Researchers have used fMRI scans to see what parts of the brain activate during creative activities. Instead of an isolated region, these studies have shown that imagination activates an extensive network of cortical and subcortical neurons throughout the brain.

This network includes the hippocampus, which you may recall is the region of the brain that is thought to control memory, especially long-term memory. This close connection between memory and imagination certainly makes sense. When we imagine something, we gather memories from the past and then rearrange them in new and creative ways.[159]

Exercising an active imagination seems likely to improve both your memory and overall cognitive health.

Something to avoid

Lisa Feldman Barrett says that one of the reasons we choose to abandon the more difficult tasks of learning is because we want a comfortable, pleasant life. I suspect that's why many people spend so much time in passive entertainment.

TV, for example, does much of the thinking for you. There's no response required from you, no need to imagine what people look like, as you would need to do with a book. No conversation, no need even to decide when to laugh. The laugh track will let you know when.

A friend of mine realized one day that she couldn't remember the names of characters on the television shows she watched—but then, why should she?

Even documentaries and so-called educational television still require little response from you, little actual effort on your part to learn something.

If you took notes, made flashcards, and then quizzed yourself, that would be beneficial. If you watched television as part of a discussion group, that would also be beneficial. But how many of us do that?

At the end of a long day, most of us want to relax in an armchair and watch our television shows or a video—and that's not helpful to our learning at all.

So my suggestion is to limit the time you spend on this entertainment and do something more active with your mind. Your brain will thank you!

What About Brain Games?

If you're looking for fun, computer games and puzzles like Sudoku or crossword puzzles are great.

But if you're looking for ways to preserve your cognitive function, these mental diversions are unlikely to have that effect. You'll get better at Sudoku, but your neural pathways will not expand. Nor will your gray matter increase.

What about those "brain games" that have become such a big business? These brain games are a $1.3

billion industry that is growing every year. But are the games worthwhile?

In a word—*no.*

If you work at these games consistently, you will become better at the games, but research has shown again and again that these benefits do not extend to your brain or your life. In fact, "an international group of 69 neuroscientists and psychologists penned an open letter to caution consumers that the claims made by the brain-game companies aren't scientifically proven."[160]

However, doesn't their research support these games? Yes, research done by the companies themselves, with too few participants to be valid. Play the games if you like them, but don't count on them to help stave off Alzheimer's.

Where to Find Learning Opportunities

1. Your local community college: Most offer lifelong learning opportunities.

2. Look for opportunities at your local library, community college, university or arts council. Local community calendars often list opportunities.

3. Join a study group at your place of worship.

4. Check out craft or fabric stores for classes.

5. Choose a topic on your own to study from history, science, literature or other topic of interest.

6. To learn a new language, check out online sources. Duolingo is a free program. (I have no financial interest in this program.)

7. If you can afford it, hire a private tutor or teacher.

8. Volunteer as a docent or guide. You will probably need to learn new content to fulfill this job.

9. If you live in a bigger city, you might check out Dabble.co, a site that lists local classes and experiences. Coursera.org and LearnThat.com offer free online courses.

A Brighter Future

Learning offers so much hope for your future! You'll enjoy the wider, richer understanding of life that learning offers. You'll gain new skills that add variety to your life, and you'll gain a sense of accomplishment. Knowledge is power!

Most of all, your brain will thrive and shine with all the new learning you give it.

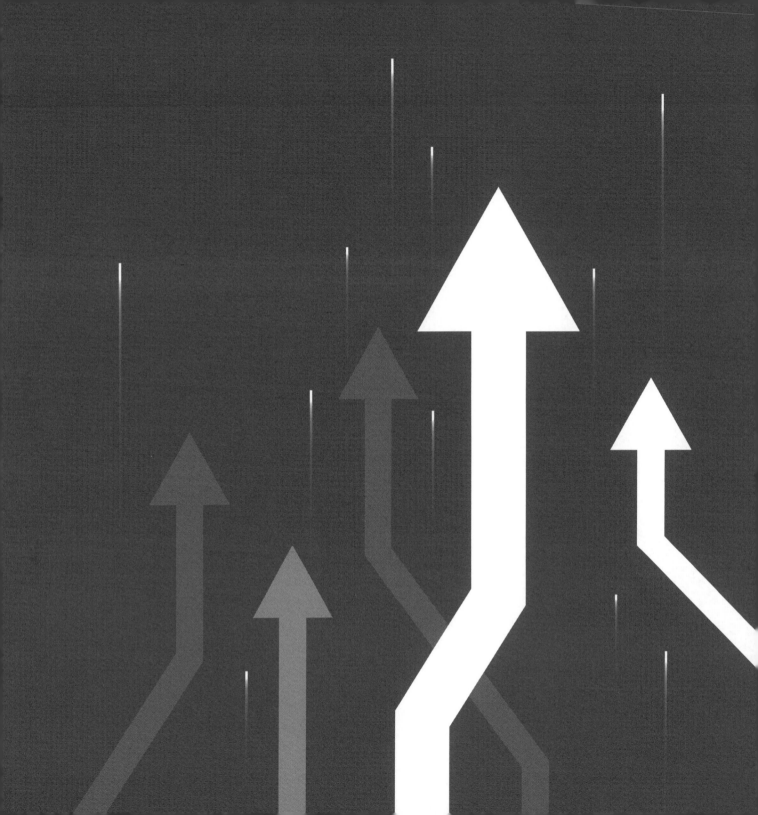

Section 4

Moving Forward

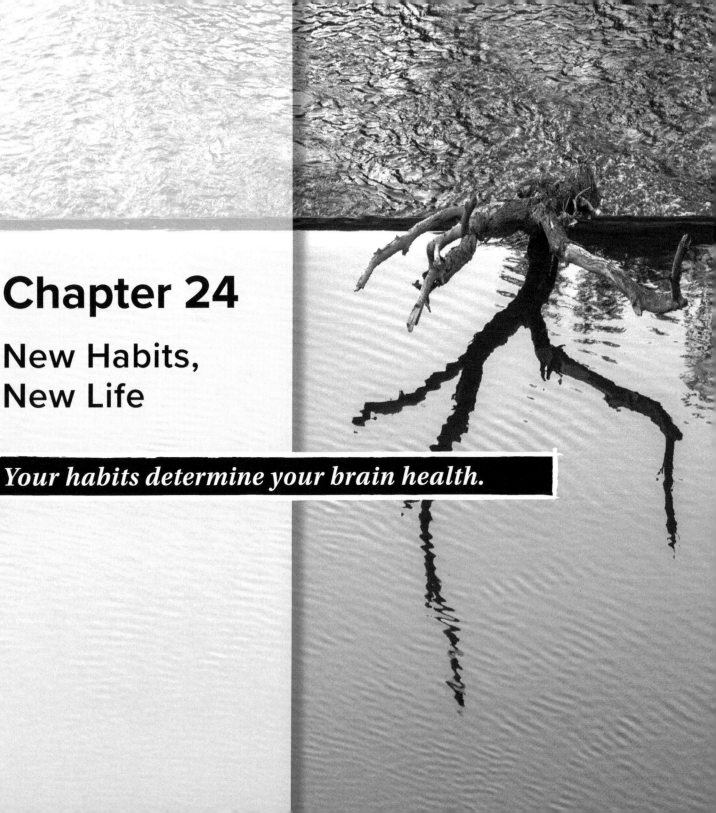

Chapter 24

New Habits, New Life

Your habits determine your brain health.

When I first tried to quit smoking, I knew I was in trouble. Breaking my habit of lighting up at every opportunity and replacing that impulse with healthy alternatives was even harder than I imagined.

So I threw myself headlong into learning everything I could about changing habits. I read books, attended conferences, consulted friends and experts and then tested everything, revised and tried again.

I successfully quit my smoking habit six years ago.

In this chapter, I will share what I learned from all these experiences. Perhaps what I learned will help you as you create your Dementia Action Plan and apply the content of this book to your own lives.

 I won't say that changing habits is easy, but for me the rewards of new, healthy habits to avoid death far exceeded the difficulty, and I think they will for you as well.

Why We Do What We Do

Most of our behavior results from two human desires:

1. We want to have joy and pleasure.

2. We want to avoid dangers, especially those that bring physical, mental and emotional pain.

We begin gathering information about these two desires almost from birth:

- No food—pain. Milk to drink—pleasure.
- Hot stove—pain. Daddy's arms—pleasure.

Each time we make choices, we reinforce a certain behavior based on these two human desires—gaining pleasure or avoiding pain.

Of course, sometimes we are confronted with conflicting desires: the pleasure of staying in a warm bed or the pleasure of the health that comes with taking a walk.

As long as we have to make a choice, we run the risk of making the unhealthier choice. In fact, our choice to do something better for our health is often quite fragile and easily set aside.

What we need is something that will predispose us to making the right choice:

In other words, a habit!

A habit is a routine of behavior that you have repeated so often that it settles into a regular, or default,

The Feedback Loop—Cue/Routine/Reward		
The Cue (whatever prompts the behavior)	**The Routine** (what you do in response to the cue)	**The Reward** (the pleasure or avoidance of pain you experience following the routine)
A stack of dirty dishes	Washing the dishes	The pleasure of a clean kitchen; avoiding the pain of seeing that dirty kitchen and having to clean it up eventually
Being given a task at work	Doing the task as soon as possible	The pleasure of a job well done and your boss's satisfaction; avoiding the pain of your boss's frustration and colleagues' complaints (whoever would have had to do the task if you didn't)
A cupcake on the counter	Not eating the cupcake	The pleasure of achieving a goal of no sugar; avoiding the pain of failing to achieve a goal, and the pain of feeling groggy from a sugar spike

tendency. Because routines predispose you to making the right decisions for your health, they are a powerful tool as you seek to improve your cognitive health.

How to Develop a New Routine

Let me start by saying it's hard to develop a routine and harder still to replace a routine with a new one. Behavioral specialists tell us the following suggestions can help.

1. **Mindfully determine what routine you want to change.**

Notice that this book does not have a step-by-step plan for the new routines you need to create. That's because the action plan you create for yourself is the best one. You know yourself better than anybody else. You know your strengths and weaknesses. You are familiar with your family and work dynamic and your health problems.

Be mindful and honest, and then think about what new routines you want to work on and in what order.

For myself, I began improving my sleep, exercising, cutting down on sugar and not smoking anymore. A friend began by improving her sleep. Another has been trying to cut down on sugar (with less success than she would like, but she keeps working on it). Still another has made multiple changes, including enrolling in a class at his community college.

The point is that you get to decide what you would like to change to make your life healthier.

2. **Figure out the feedback loop for the behavior you want to become a routine.**

For each behavior, there's a feedback loop that includes a cue, a routine behavior and a reward. To change your current routine, you'll need to change either the cue or the reward (or both).

Let's consider each element of the feedback loop in a little more detail.

The cue: Every behavior has a cue. This event causes the impulse or decision that leads to the routine behavior.

You already have many cues in your life. It could be the alarm going off in the morning. That usually starts some routine behaviors. Sitting down at your desk in the morning arouses the desire for a hot cup of coffee.

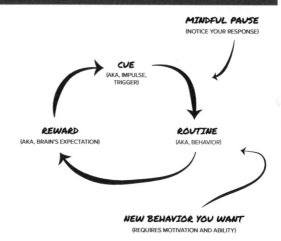

HOW HABITS WORK

Our lives have many routines. All of them involve a circular pattern of cues, routines and rewards.

Coming home from work triggers the desire for a quick snack. End-of-the-day weariness provokes a desire to lie down on the couch and watch TV.

As you have been reading this book, perhaps a desire for a vibrant, functioning brain has awakened a generalized desire for a healthier lifestyle. Now comes the hard part—figuring out the best cues for each change you want to make.

What can serve as a cue to turn off screens an hour before bed so that you can get to sleep easier? What can

Page 211

cause you to eat fruit after dinner instead of ice cream? What can be a cue for you to spend your dinner time talking to your spouse rather than watching TV?

As you create your personalized *Dementia Action Plan*, these are questions you'll need to answer if you want to change your routines.

The habits you want to develop: These are the specific goals you set for your life, one by one. Be realistic and set goals you believe you can do again and again.

If you want to introduce more movement into your life, for example, instead of making your goal 10,000 steps a day, break that big goal into smaller behaviors that are practical and enjoyable. Start by walking to the mailbox every day and work up from there.

Make it a break from work or chores around the house if you can. That will become another reward for the new behavior. Add another short walk in the evening after dinner.

As you walk more and more, you'll find other rewards in this healthy behavior, and it will soon become a habit.

These are just suggestions, of course. The key is to set your own practical and achievable goals.

Reward: This is the most powerful component of the feedback loop. This part—deciding what will inspire and reinforce the change you want to make—needs to be strong enough to motivate the good behavior again

and again until it becomes a new habit for you.

The strength of a reward depends on an individual person's perspective. To some, the reward of a good night's sleep will be enough to motivate a regular sleep schedule. For others, giving up a late night on Friday requires a better reward. The point is the right reward is one that will motivate you.

Unfortunately, there's always a gap between the new routine and the reward for healthier choices. In the short term, a walk this morning robs you of sleep and may even make you feel sore. Only when you do it consistently for a month or two do you get the reward of feeling so much better. The same with sugar. Refuse that cupcake, and in the short term your craving continues to gnaw at you. Only with time do those sugar cravings recede and eventually disappear.

In my own life, 90 days is an optimal length of time. When I got up and walked for 90 days, I felt so much better that I actually enjoyed getting up early enough to walk before work. Limiting processed foods, going to bed earlier, meditating—do anything for 90 days, and maybe, like me, you won't want to stop.

3. **Once you have a plan for a new feedback loop, try it out for a week or two.**

With every new routine there's always a moment when you ask yourself, *Will I or won't I?* In that moment, think first what is throwing up a roadblock to your new habit. Is it an ignorance of how to meditate? A concern about weeds in your lawn? Something on TV that made you crave something sweet? Address issues like these, and your progress toward a new habit should improve.

Next, think about how to strengthen your reward. I have a friend who imagines her granddaughter in a wedding dress. Other times, she thinks of being of sound mind during her later years and being able to enjoy time with her husband (as opposed to him having to take care of her when she is there only in body). A shorter-term reward is her children's appreciation for the changes she has made.

This doesn't necessarily make saying no to cookies easier, but she says these rewards do always convince her to get back on track. Stack the rewards in your favor.

If necessary, revise your goal. Smaller steps make the journey longer, but you will still get there!

Two Examples

Exercising

This is an important goal for your brain, and it's a positive new routine you can develop. Please remember, however, to speak with your doctor before starting any new exercise routine.

1. *Cue:* What can be the event in your life that results in exercise? Take some time to think about this. Perhaps you are meeting a friend to walk your dogs. Perhaps it can be a mid-morning break from your desk. Perhaps it's a time of day or a certain place that cues your commitment to exercise.

2. *Behavior:* You have many options for exercise. Choose one that you enjoy enough to do it again and again, or choose a variety of methods. Start small and add to your goal. If you like nature, walk outside. If you like company, join an exercise class. For your brain, it's best to include interval and strength training, but to begin, do what you enjoy.

3. *Reward:* Long-term rewards don't tend to motivate immediate changes in behavior. Can you think of something right away that will reward you? It might be a break from work. Or the pleasure or sense of accomplishment you feel or the general good feeling you get after you have pushed yourself. (Those are probably endorphins.) Eventually, you'll start getting the longer-term rewards like easier breathing, less weight, stronger muscles, and wow, what a payoff!

Eating less added sugar

This is a hard one because the typical reward for sugar is a release of dopamine, the feel-good hormone in your brain. Sugar becomes an addiction. We get a hit of sugar, and as soon as the dopamine wears off we want some more—especially in times of stress, loneliness or sorrow.

Some people find that they have to eliminate sugar from their diet entirely to be able to control their addiction to sweets. However, if you think you can control your desire for sugar by changing your routines, here are some suggestions:

1. *Cue:* Over the course of a week or two, take careful notes about when you feel a craving for sugar. It might be after a heavy meal at lunch or perhaps when someone brings sweets to the coffee room. For many, it occurs in the evening as they watch TV. Then ask yourself how you can change this cue. Don't go to the coffee room? Avoid heavy lunches? Stop watching TV, or at least get rid of the sweets you want to eat in front of the TV?

2. *Behavior:* The new routine you want to establish is vitally important to eating less added sugar because something needs to replace what sugar is providing. Research has indicated that a snack high in protein and good fats can be an excellent substitute. So consider making a snack of nuts your new routine or some roasted chickpeas. In the evening, perhaps your new routine can be eating a piece of low-glycemic fruit like an apple. This healthy snack offers a sweet flavor packaged with fiber and many nutrients.

3. *Reward:* Long-term, you are doing good for your brain. Short-term, enjoy the satisfaction of keeping your goal. Some accountability can also help. Start a DWS Club (Down With Sugar), or perhaps a friend will serve as an accountability coach. With sugar, you will not have to get through many days before you start feeling so much better.

Moving Forward

You now know many ways to reduce your risk of Alzheimer's dementia.

Cognitive decline doesn't just happen in your brain. Instead, many structures in your body affect the ability of your brain to function well: mitochondria, small to large organs, neurotransmitters, inflammation, infection, sleep, nutrition, stress, as well as your emotional and spiritual health.

Your brain and neurons need to work together and function well to avoid Alzheimer's. But so do the other parts of your body, protected by sleep and proper nutrition.

You have to live well; avoid anger, stress, anxiety, resentment, and isolation; and seek opportunities for joy, laughter, love, and physical and emotional connections with others.

If you can do this, you can improve not only your life but the lives of your family and community.

Here, at the end of this book, I am impressed again with this one fact: Dementia is not a simple disease with a quick and easy treatment.

Imagine that you were my patient, coming to me with concerns about Alzheimer's. Knowing what I know now, I would reject a simple diagnosis of Alzheimer's because the label would tempt me to take shortcuts and offer solutions that are easy for me to propose, but would not work well for you.

Instead, I would learn about your family and connections, your jobs and hobbies, your fears, passions and abilities.

Most of all, I would want to learn what might motivate you to make the changes that would improve your cognitive health. Only then could I begin to propose solutions that would enhance your life.

Throughout this book, I have suggested ways to reduce your risk of Alzheimer's dementia. I hope you will develop your plan of action, and that as you carry out that plan, you will achieve a more vibrant, healthy and joyful life.

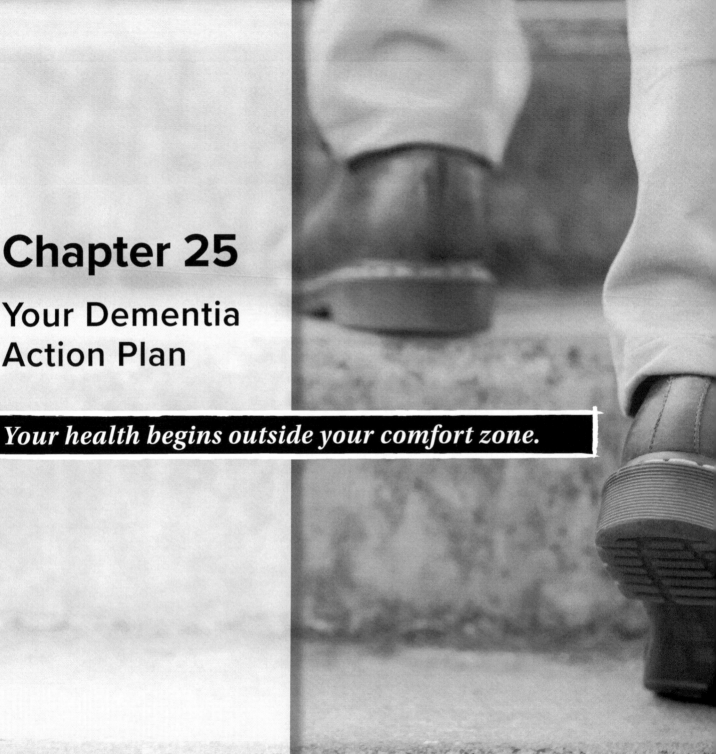

Chapter 25

Your Dementia Action Plan

Your health begins outside your comfort zone.

We now come to the ultimate purpose of this book—your own, personalized Dementia Action Plan for reducing your risk of Alzheimer's dementia.

For many of you, the information in this book is not new to you. Bookstores are stocked with books about nutrition, the benefits of exercise, how to reduce stress and much more about healthy living.

When it comes to healthier living, there's a tsunami of confusing information available on TV and social media, advertisements and the Internet.

But knowing does not always change behavior. We know what to do and still don't do it. We know what not to do, and we still keep repeating it. We keep stressing out, sleeping poorly, choosing not to exercise and eating junk foods. We hurt ourselves in countless ways every day.

What will make us willing to exchange the pleasures of another 30 minutes in bed for a 30-minute walk? How can we choose healthy soup instead of chicken wings or an apple instead of a brownie?

Based on my own experiences, combined with a concerted effort to sort out what works and what doesn't, I offer the following principles which I believe will be of use to you.

Know your why

Two people refuse dessert. One says, "I'm giving up sweets because I'm going to Florida and want to look good in my swimsuit." The other says, "I've given up sweets to protect my brain."

The first person is giving up something for a short-term gain. The second is changing his or her future. As you make your Dementia Action Plan, embrace the scope of your goals and their life-changing impact.

Expand your comfort zone

As we grow, based on our family dynamics, our culture and society, we make choices about how we will behave. We choose these behaviors because they either give us pleasure or they remove pain and suffering.

At first, these choices are as fragile as a spider web. Over time, as we repeat the choices again and again, they become habits. We do them without thinking. Even our cravings become habitual.

If you want to develop new habits, you will need to be very intentional about your choices. Your behavior will be fragile at this point. Because you are not used to these choices, each one will push you out of your comfort zone.

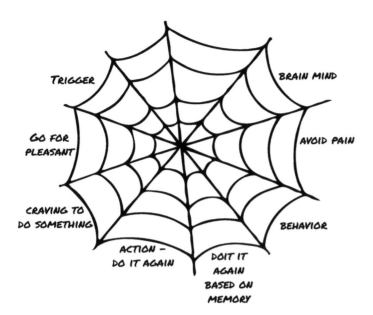

Labels on the web (clockwise from top): BRAIN MIND, AVOID PAIN, BEHAVIOR, DO IT AGAIN BASED ON MEMORY, ACTION – DO IT AGAIN, CRAVING TO DO SOMETHING, GO FOR PLEASANT, TRIGGER

New behaviors can seem as fragile as a spider web.

But if you take advantage of each opportunity to make this new choice, over time, your behavior will become a habit, and a new, healthier comfort zone will develop.

Savor the journey

Keep your eye on the prize, we tell each other, but the journey itself can be beautiful—especially as you embark on a journey toward better health.

Each victory along the way will bring its own pleasures. Something as small as getting up a little earlier to exercise will change the way you feel about yourself through that day. You set a goal. You followed through. That says something good about who you are.

In this way, you'll reap not only physical rewards but also emotional and spiritual rewards along the way. So embrace the small victories. Revel in them!

As you change your life, you'll also find pleasure in unexpected places. That early-morning walk? You may end up craving it. The apple instead of ice cream? You'll be surprised at the pleasure it can bring you.

Look for the pleasure inherent in each new habit. Pleasure is pleasure, and your body will thrive as you give it more of what it needs.

Make a plan

By now, you know that protecting your memory and improving your cognitive function is a complex issue. To succeed, you need a plan.

In this book, I have given you information about how you can reduce your risk of Alzheimer's dementia and protect your memory. In this chapter, I will provide a framework for you to prepare a personalized Dementia Action Plan to help make that happen.

Creating Your Dementia Action Plan

Preparation: Willpower

Before you pick up pen and paper to write out your plan, do yourself a favor, and pause. Give yourself time to decide if you are ready for these changes.

Why have you been reading this book? Are you concerned about your memory? Is something driving you to reduce your risk of Alzheimer's dementia?

If you don't really think anything is wrong, you are not ready. If someone else is concerned about you and wants you to make changes, again, you are not ready. Trust me. You need to do this for yourself because *you* make the choice, not someone else.

Even if you know you have a problem, but you don't want to make changes now, again you are not ready.

Emotional Outlook

Think of your emotional outlook as a load-bearing wall that will reinforce and fortify every aspect of your Dementia Action Plan. Do you have any resentment, anger or fear that could weaken your efforts? Seek a way to set these aside.

At the same time, mindfully consider the love, forgiveness and kindness you can give yourself and others. Make a list of your own strongest qualities. These positive emotions will inspire and motivate you, especially when you encounter inevitable setbacks.

Education: Skillpower

If you are concerned for yourself, if you know you need help, and you're ready to do what's necessary today, then you've taken your first step to memory improvement and cognitive health.

This book has lots of information to absorb, and I hope you have found it useful and informative. If you have taken time to gather your own motivations,

routines and social support, and if you feel confident about your understanding of dementia and the seven modifiable lifestyle changes, there's still one more thing you can do—a self assessment related to each of these lifestyle changes.

In a very relaxed way (no judgment!), think about your current behaviors. This will help you know what to emphasize in your plan.

Sleep: Do you regularly get 7-8 hours of sleep without long interruptions? Do you generally get to sleep easily and wake up at the same time each day?

Movement: How often do you move during the day? At work, do you sit most of the day? Do you have a long commute? Do you spend any time outside in the sunshine? If you regularly exercise, what time of day do you do it? Do you vary the kind of exercise you get?

Nutrition: How many servings of vegetables do you eat each day? How many servings of fruit? What kind of oil do you use? Do you ever eat beans and legumes (such as lentils)? How many processed foods do you eat during the week (anything prepared somewhere else)? Fast food? Foods with added sugar?

You may also want to do a pantry purge of foods you know will trip you up such as desserts, soft drinks, juices and processed foods.

Stress: Do you find it hard to relax? Do you have a generalized sense of concern most of the time?

Illness ←————————→ Wellness

Are your muscles often tight? Do you wake up at 4:00 in the morning and have trouble getting back to sleep because you are worrying? Does your forehead have a constant furrow? Are your shoulders constantly hunched? Is your blood pressure a problem?

Clean water, air, and environment: How do you get most of your hydration? How many soft drinks and fruit juices do you drink each day? If you drink water, is it unfiltered tap or well water? How much alcohol do you drink each day?

Do you filter your air? Do live near a freeway or a heavily traveled road? Do you smoke or live with someone who does? Do you have concerns about mold in your home?

Consider your cleaning supplies and personal care products. Do they have the toxins listed in Chapter 19? How about your lawn care or garden products? Do you use any pesticides? Have you considered your stance on fluoride, electromagnetic fields, tobacco and alcohol? Perhaps it's time to request a medication review from your doctor.

A fairly simple step you can take: Purchase a filtration device for your air and water. Check the Interact Well Care website for suggestions.

Relationships: How would you assess your social contacts? Do you spend time with other people in a social setting? Do you often feel lonely, even

in a crowd? Are you challenging your brain by learning something new?

It might be helpful to gather your loved ones together, especially your partner, and explain what you are doing. Your partner may be willing to join you on this health adventure (I hope so), and if your friends and family know what you are doing, they can encourage you.

Best of all would be an accountability partner, someone you can check in with regularly to report your successes and challenges. You may also consider a coach for your journey.

Sensory and Mental Stimulation: Do you need an eye or ear check-up? Does aromatherapy as a means of calming your stress appeal to you? Do you need to quit smoking, which harms your sense of taste? Would you consider receiving regular massages? As for learning, what subject or skill could you invest in—a new instrument, cooking, yoga, chess? Find something that will challenge you.

As you think through these questions, remember that there's a continuum between illness and wellness.

On some of these lifestyle choices, you may be toward Wellness on the continuum. Perhaps you have an excellent exercise program, or you already eat a diet with no added sugar.

Perhaps instead, like I was, you are much closer to Illness. I smoked, got terrible sleep, barely moved at all,

Your Dementia Action Plan

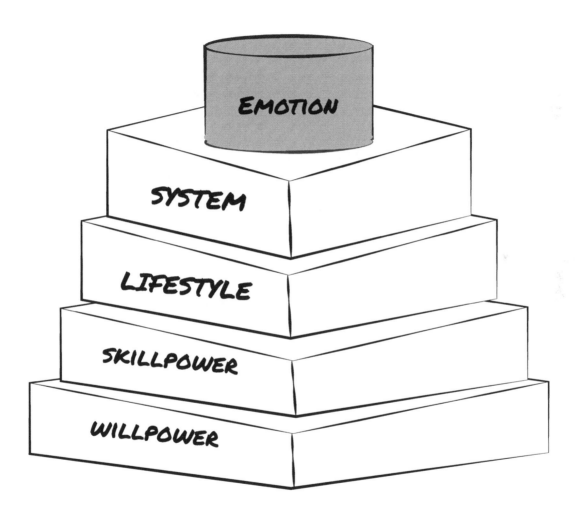

Remember, these are not sequential steps. Your emotional outlook supports everything you do, and you will undoubtedly move back and forth among the other stages.

was addicted to sugary cereal and drank diet soft drinks obsessively.

Wherever you are on this continuum, it's okay! You have the power to improve your health. Your body will help you. It wants to thrive.

Modifiable Lifestyle Changes

Once you have had some time to consider your lifestyle choices, it's time to prepare for your action plan. This is the time for pencil and paper (or your computer, if you prefer). For your action plan, you'll need to identify 90-day goals and weekly steps.

You can work on as many of the seven modifiable lifestyle changes as you want, but keep the weekly steps small so that you can experience victories each week.

You can download helpful forms from InteractWellCare.com to help make this part of your plan.

90-day goals and weekly steps

Everything in your health is connected in some way. Your exercise affects your stress levels. Better stress levels will allow you to sleep better. Healthy food will affect how much you can exercise, and better sleep will improve everything. So whichever of the seven modifiable risk factors you choose to work on first, the others will benefit as well.

Even so, I recommend that you address sleep first. If you are not getting enough sleep, everything

is suffering. Sleep is your first line of defense against Alzheimer's because during sleep your brain is cleansed. If you can improve your sleep, everything else will be easier to accomplish. The chapter on sleep explains many ways that you can improve your sleep. I recommend two important first steps: Turn screens off an hour before bedtime and try to go to sleep and get up at the same time every day.

For food, your 90-day goal may be to eat fewer processed foods. Your smaller step might be to pre-make lunches for the week, such as salads or soups.

For "exercise," your 90-day goal might be to walk 30 minutes each day. Your smaller step might be to walk to the end of the block and back.

For stress, your 90-day goal might be to meditate every day. Your small step could be to increase the time you spend in natural light. Sunlight early in the morning awakens you for the day and twilight calms you for the evening.

For social relationships, your 90-day goal might be to meet with a friend every week. Your small step could be to invite a friend for a walk this week.

For sensory and mental stimulation, your 90-day goal may be to learn more about World War II. Your small step might be to read a biography of Churchill.

These are just ideas, of course. You know the goals you need and what will help you best. And you know how many of the modifiable risk factors you want to work on at a time.

If you stick with your 90-day plan to improve your sleep, activity level, nutrition, stress and relationships, you will be ready to dig deeper into the other topics covered in this book. These include further detoxifying your life, improving your gut health, mitochondria, and hormone imbalances, eliminating endocrine disruptors and the other topics discussed in this book. We include instructions in each chapter.

I suggest you use the same 90-day, small-step format to address these other topics.

Monitoring your progress

If you like to keep track of things, you can use the downloadable form from InteractWellCare.com to check off good days. Put this form where your partner or family members can see it. However, if you absolutely detest keeping track of things (I know you're out there!), perhaps you could track your progress once a week even in just general terms.

Journaling offers an excellent way to be mindful during this journey. By marking important victories and struggles, you will have a diagram to look back at when you meet obstacles. Surprisingly, journaling will also decrease your stress because it allows you to frame your experiences in a coherent way.

An accountability partner can also help monitor and inspire your progress. We all need encouragement. Perhaps a son or daughter could text you every couple of days for an update, or a friend could call once a week. These human connections are so powerful!

Corrections

Inevitably, you will need to modify your plan at some point. This is completely natural. Your journey will have many side trips, recalculations and corrections.

More than likely, you will find yourself unable to begin a new behavior or to stop an unwanted behavior. In either case, for a few days continue as things are. This will give you a chance to do a trigger-behavior-reward analysis. (The previous chapter describes these three aspects of any behavior.)

Understanding what is triggering a behavior and the consequences of that behavior will empower a new approach.

Cues: First, play close attention to what triggers an unwanted behavior.

That soft drink you have mid-morning? Perhaps you are just bored, and a quick walk outside will break the monotony. Checking your device while in bed? You can change that trigger by leaving your device in the kitchen on vibrate. Sleeping in instead of exercising? Perhaps you aren't getting enough sleep.

If you can correctly identify your triggers, you will have more control over the behavior that follows.

Rewards: Addiction clinics understand the value of taking time to consider the behavior, especially in light of its rewards.

These clinics tell people who want to quit smoking to keep smoking for a few more days. If people pay attention to the whole experience—when they make the purchase, when they light up, inhale and exhale, and also how smoking smells, tastes and feels—they usually begin noticing the downsides of the cigarettes.

When I really paid attention to my smoking, I noticed how much my eyes stung from the smoke. I realized my breath always smelled like tobacco and that the taste never completely left my mouth. I began to find smoking very unattractive. My "rewards" began to feel like punishments.

In the clinics, people are then advised to think about how their lives will be better when they stop smoking—better breathing, richer flavors, respect from family and friends, money for other pursuits. These were the new and better rewards that motivated me.

I'm not going to say I didn't relapse. But when I did smoke another cigarette, I had a much bigger understanding of what was happening.

You know yourself better than anybody else. You know your strengths and weaknesses. You know your habits and behaviors and cravings.

If you are having trouble following through on a goal, non-judgmentally pay attention to what you are feeling, doing and choosing as you engage in that behavior. Then revise your trigger or reward to make the new, healthier behavior more possible.

System Changes

As you address your modifiable lifestyle changes, you will find that your body's systems and organs respond with greater health.

- Your hormones will become more balanced.
- Your cells' mitochondria will provide more energy.
- Your immune system will become more effective.
- Your gut will function better.
- Your bones and muscles will become stronger.
- Your heart will become more powerful.

Maintenance

Whatever steps you take, small or big, you'll want to stick with them, because the real value of your Dementia Action Plan comes in this phase—the maintenance phase.

As you progress toward this stage, inevitably you will encounter relapses, setbacks and the need to revise goals and motivations. Changing a behavior into a new and better routine is rarely a straight line. Some people are very strong, with great self-control. They make an action plan, and they stick to it. That's great for them!

I am definitely not one of those people. My road is always bumpy, with lots of twists and turns. If that's true for you, that's okay as long as you keep moving forward. At the end of the day, as long as you are moving toward your goals—however unevenly—and your overall progress is positive, that's all you need.

Eventually, your new and better lifestyle choices will become a routine, choices you make without having to think about them. You're solid!

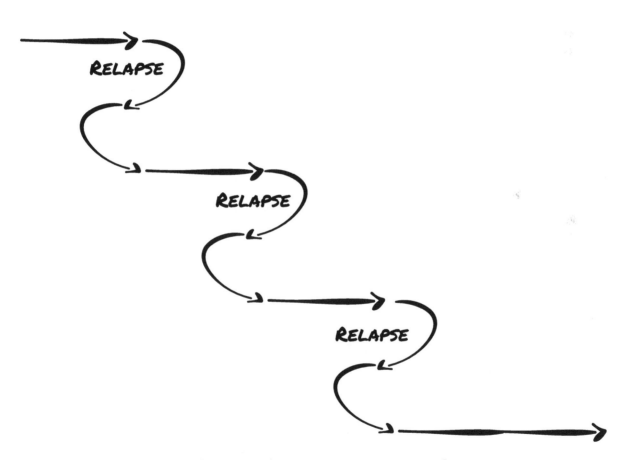

Typical progress for any Dementia Action Plan—
It's a journey!

A Salute to Caregivers

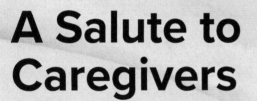

"Caregivers are often the casualities, the hidden victims. No one sees the sacrifices they make."

- Judith L. London

Dear Caregiver,

If you feel that I have ignored your long-time role and sacrifices, I sincerely apologize. Your daily care for a person living with Alzheimer's is essential. Thank you for everything you do.

The circle of life. It's a cold, hard reality. Our mothers, fathers or other loved ones raised us. From the minute we came into this world, they fed us, protected us, bathed us and dressed us. They taught us to walk and talk. They taught us to love and feel compassion. They taught us to treat others as we want them to treat us. They loved us unconditionally and without any restraint.

Eventually, the tables turn. Our parents and loved ones need us. For some of us, our parents need us to remind them to take their medication, to eat, dress and bathe. Some of us become responsible for our parents' safety.

As a caregiver, you often have to put your loved one's needs above your own and even above the needs of your own family.

Cognitive impairment in all its forms changes the lives of caregivers like you. Typically, caregivers lose touch with family and friends. They are often among the hidden and forgotten people at the center of the ugly cage of memory loss. Most caregivers do their job at a high cost financially, physically, emotionally and spiritually.

In 2016 alone, family and friends provided more than ***20 billion hours of unpaid care*** to people with some cognitive impairment. Women provided most of that care.

Someone who has not experienced any kind of caregiving to a person with cognitive impairment cannot really imagine how hard this job is—the endless days and nights, the building anxiety, the deep sorrow of seeing your mom or dad forget who you are, the exhaustion of having parents argue with you about what they need to do. They slip away in every respect except physically. Even if you are not crying, you are grieving.

But there's an even more substantial burden that many caregivers must carry.

If we take care of loved ones after open heart surgery or knee replacement or even cancer and chemotherapy, it can be physically and emotionally exhausting. But as we help them, they are still with us. They smile, thank us, respond to us in familiar ways, and we have hope that they can get better. Sadly, the circumstances involving Alzheimer's dementia differ substantially.

When you care for your loved ones with Alzheimer's, you are taking care of two people—the parent who still lives in your memory and the one whom your parent is becoming. Increasingly, you mourn the person who loved and cared for you, but at the same time, you must care for a person who doesn't know you and may even resent you. You are helpless in the face of this horrible disease, and inevitably guilt moves into your house like a bad smell.

Worst of all, you have no hope that things will ever get better, only worse.

Children become increasingly independent. Your loved one with Alzheimer's becomes less and less so. The day comes when you can no longer leave your loved one alone. You will no longer go to the store without arranging care for them. Vacations are a thing of the past—a memory of a happier time. Often, your loved one becomes more agitated and increasingly violent. You never know what your loved one's mood will be from day to day.

One day, you will realize that you can no longer take care of your mom or dad. You already keep the door locked so they cannot go out on their own. You have taken every step you can to eliminate dangers inside your home.

But now your loved one feels threatened and has become increasingly aggressive. You have to be with them continually, and it's hard to find time to go to the bathroom without putting them at risk. You are becoming sleep deprived because of the demands of caregiving and the added stress is a terrible burden.

And so you arrange for your loved one to move into assisted care or a nursing facility. The day when you walk away from the facility, knowing that your loved one will not be leaving with you, is often devastating. Many caregivers feel like they have failed.

If you are lucky enough, you may know the physician at the facility or one of the staff members. Knowing that someone at the facility is on your side helps a little with the guilt. Even so, at the nursing facility, your loved one will not have their pets, furnishings or familiar surroundings. The rooms they now use are different, as is the glass they use for drinking water, the mattress they sleep on and the many unfamiliar faces. This makes them deteriorate faster and faster.

Eventually, with Alzheimer's, your loved one will forget everything—to eat, to drink, even to swallow, and ultimately, they will forget to breathe. Then the long goodbye will end. So much loss!

If you are a caregiver, I suspect you have already thought about legal and financial plans, about long-term care and government support. I will not cover any of these, nor will I suggest a plan of care, because as the caregiver, it will be primarily up to you to devise a plan of care for your loved one.

But I do want to remind you to take care of yourself as you care for your loved one. In fact, for the sake of your loved one, *take care of yourself first*. In airplanes, the flight attendant says to put your oxygen mask on first and only then to help your loved ones. You need to care first for your own physical, emotional and spiritual health if you want to keep meeting the needs of your loved one.

In particular, *you must take care of your cognitive health* during this difficult time. Think of all that the task of caregiving has brought into your life—anxiety, stress, inactivity, lack of sleep and exercise, and often less than adequate nutrition.

All these increase your risk of Alzheimer's. If you fail to care for yourself today, you may be the one who needs a caregiver tomorrow.

You are not alone. There are people in your community who want to help, who understand what you are facing and who are willing to give of their time and love to help you through the nightmare you are experiencing.

We are witnessing history. A pill or effective treatment is still in the future. For now, for the sake of our families and our communities, we must all work together to do what we can to defeat the loss that comes from Alzheimer's.

And that includes doing all you can to avoid your own risk of Alzheimer's.

I sincerely wish you all the best.

Hamid Reza Sagha

Endnotes

1 You can check these and other statistics about Alzheimer's at these three websites: Alzheimer's Association. What is dementia? Retrieved December 31, 2018 from https://www.alz.org/alzheimers-dementia/what-is-dementia; National Institute on Aging (2019, August 1). Alzheimer's Disease Fact Sheet. Retrieved from https://www.nia.nih.gov/health/alzheimers-disease-fact-sheet; Alzheimer's Statistics (2017). Retrieved from https://www.alzheimers.net/resources/alzheimers-statistics/

2 What is a neuron? (2018, July 4). Retrieved from https://qbi.uq.edu.au/brain/brain-anatomy/what-neuron

3 Azvolinsky, A. (2016, May). Amyloid thwarts microbial invaders. Retrieved from https://www.the-scientist.com/daily-news/amyloid-thwarts-microbial-invaders-33485

4 For more information see O'Brien, R. J. & Wong, P. C. (2011). Amyloid precursor protein processing & Alzheimer's disease. Annual Review of Neuroscience, 34, 185-204.

5 NewCenter. Scientists reveal how beta-amyloid may cause Alzheimer's. Retrieved from https://med.stanford.edu/news/all-news/2013/09/scientists-reveal-how-beta-amyloid-may-cause-alzheimers.html

6 Siegenthaler, B.M., & Rajendran, L. (2016, February 16). Gamma secretase regulates alpha secretase cleavage of the Alzheimer's disease, amyloid precursor protein. Retrieved from https://sciencematters.io/articles/201601000003

7 New Alzheimer's therapy shows promise in reducing plaques in brain. (2016, September). Retrieved from https://alzheimersnewstoday.com/2016/09/07/alzheimers-investigational-drug-reduces-brain-amyloid-plaques/

8 For more information on tau tangles, see AbbVie (2017, June 29). The tangled web of tau. https://www.youtube.com/watch?v=AV1BqpOyHmM

9 Facts and Figures. (2019, March 5). Alzheimer's Association, Retrieved from https://www.alz.org/alzheimers-dementia/facts-figures

10 For a lengthier but still straightforward description of the immune system, I highly recommend Khan Academy's Immunology videos; for B cells and T cells, I especially recommend the video on B cells. Retrieved from https://www.khanacademy.org/science/biology/human-biology/immunology/v/b-lymphocytes-b-cells

11 Nordqvist, C. (2017, November 24). Everything you need to know about inflammation. Retrieved from https://www.medicalnewstoday.com/articles/248423.php

12 Kipnis, J. (2018, August). The seventh sense. Scientific American, 33.

13 Kipnis, J. (2018, August). The seventh sense. Scientific American, 33.

14 Neuroinflammation in Alzheimer's disease. (2015, March 16). Retrieved from https://www.sciencedirect.com/science/article/abs/pii/S1474442215700165

15 Daneman, R. & Prat, A. (2015). The blood-brain barrier. Cold Spring Harbor Perspectives in Biology, 7(1).

16 For an excellent, more in-depth description of inflammation and Alzheimer's disease, see Rubio-Perez, J.M. & Morillas-Ruiz, J.M. (2012). A review: Inflammatory process in Alzheimer's disease, role of cytokine. Retrieved from https://www.ncbi.nlm.nih.gov/pmc/articles/PMC3330269/

17 Perry, V.H. & Teeling, J. (2013). Microglia & macrophages of the central nervous system: The contribution of microglia priming and systemic inflammation to chronic neurodegeneration. Seminars in immunopathology, 35(5), 601-612.

18 Graff-Rodford, J. (2017, March 29). Early onset Alzheimer's: When symptoms begin before age 65. Retrieved from https://mayoclinic.org/diseases-conditions/alzheimers-disease/in-depth/alzheimer s/art-20048356

19 Keshavan, M. (2017, August 22). At high risk for Alzheimer's, they're experimenting on themselves. Retrieved from https://statnews.com/2017/08/22/alzheimers-apoe4-risk/

20 Hayasaki, E. (2018, May 15). Identical twins hint at how environments change gene expression. Retrieved from https://www.theatlantic.com/science/archive/2018/05/twin-epigenetics/560189/

21 Miller, P. (2012, January). A thing or two about twins. Retrieved from https://www.nationalgeographic.com/magazine/2012/01/identical-twins-science-dna-portraits/

22 Miller, P. (2012, January). A thing or two about twins. Retrieved from https://www.nationalgeographic.com/magazine/2012/01/identical-twins-science-dna-portraits/

23 These neurotransmitters are probably keeping you up at night. (2016, October 5). Neuroscientist Colin Gerber provides this information in an answer via Quora. Retrieved from https://www.forbes.com/sites/quora/2016/10/05/these-neurotransmitters-are-probably-keeping-you-up-at-night/#661359bd12238

24 Hurtado-Alvarado, G., Dominguez-Salazar, E., Pavon, L., Velazquez-Moctezuma, J. & Gomez-Gonzalez, B. (2016, August). Blood-brain barrier description induced by chronic sleep loss: Low-grade inflammation may be the link. Retrieved from http://dx.doi.org/10.1155/2016/4576012

25 Definition of glial cell. Retrieved from https://www.medicinenet.com/script/main/art.asp?articlekey=11382

26 How sleep clears the brain. (2013, October 28). Retrieved from https://www.nih.gov/news-events/nih-research-matters/how-sleep-clears-brain

27 Some people are able to stop using the CPAP machine if they lose enough weight. That happened to me.

28 Brubaker, M. (2017, January 12). Exercise...it does a body good: 20 minutes can act as anti-inflammatory. Retrieved from https://ucsdnews.ucsd.edu/pressrelease/exercise_it_does_a_body_good_20_minutes_can_act_as_anti_inflammatory

29 The brain has other neurotrophins, but BDNF seems to be the most important.

30 BDNF gene: Brain-derived neurotrophic factor. Retrieved from https://ghr.nlm.nih.gov/gene/BDNF

31 Qtd. in Dahl, M. (2015, April). How exercise may protect against Alzheimer's. Retrieved from https://www.thecut.com/2015/04/how-exercise-may-protect-against-alzheimers.html

32 Longevity hormone boosts memory and protects brain from aging in mice. (2017, August). Retrieved from https://www.sciencedaily.com/releases/2017/08/170808150006.htm

33 Matsubara, T., Miyaki, A., Akazawa, N., Choi, Y., Ra, S.G., Tanahashi, K., Kumagi, H., Oikawa, S., Maeda, S. (2013, December). Aerobic exercise training increases plasma klotho levels and reduces arterial stiffness in postmenopausal women. Retrieved from https://www.ncbi.nlm.nih.gov/pubmed/24322608

34 Bergland, C. (2017, July). One more reason aerobic exercise is so good for your brain. Retrieved from https://www.psychologytoday.com/us/blog/the-athletes-way/201707/one-more-reason-aerobic-exercise-is-so-good-your-brain

35 Robinson, M.M., et al. (2017, March). Enhanced protein translation underlies improved metabolic and physical adaptations to different exercise training modes in young and old humans. Retrieved from https://www.cell.com/cell-metabolism/fulltext/S1550-4131(17)30099-2

36 Mayo Clinic Staff. Strength training: Get stronger, leaner, healthier. Retrieved from https://www.mayoclinic.org/healthy-lifestyle/fitness/in-depth/strength-training/art-20046670

37 You can also find simple instructions here: Henderzahs-Mason, J.M. Balance training: Boost your long-term health with these exercises. https://www.mayoclinic.org/healthy-lifestyle/fitness/in-depth/balance-training-to-boost-health/art-20270119

38 What are mitochondria? (1970, November 7). Retrieved from http://www.mrc-mbu.cam.ac.uk/what-are-mitochondria

39 Villines, Z. Free radicals: How do they affect the body? Retrieved from https://www.medicalnewstoday.com/articles/318652.php

40 Walton, A. G. (2012, August 30). How much sugar are Americans eating? Retrieved from https://www.forbes.com/sites/alicegwalton/2012/08/30/how-much-sugar-are-americans-eating-infographic/#6ecf3f2b4ee7

41 Walton, A. G. (2012, August 30). How much sugar are Americans eating? Retrieved from https://www.forbes.com/sites/alicegwalton/2012/08/30/how-much-sugar-are-americans-eating-infographic/#6ecf3f2b4ee7

42 Gregory, A. (2017, February 23). Dementia could be triggered by eating too much sugar, landmark study reveals. Retrieved from http://www.mirror.co.uk/science/dementia-could-triggered-eating-much-9904672

43 Holford, P. (2015, August 24). How sugar ages the brain. Retrieved from https://www.patrickholford.com/advice/how-sugar-ages-brain

44 Calandra, T. & Roger, T. (2002, October 1). Macrophage migration inhibitory factor: A regulator of innate immunity. Retrieved from https://www.ncbi.nlm.nih.gov/pubmed/14502271

45 Holford, P. (2015, August 24). How sugar ages the brain. Retrieved from https://www.patrickholford.com/advice/how-sugar-ages-brain

46 Type 3 diabetes: Symptoms, treatment, causes and more. Retrieved from https://www.healthline.com/health/type-3-diabetes

47 Kaplan, K. (2011, September 20). Diabetes increases the risk of dementia and Alzheimer's disease. Retrieved from http://articles.latimes.com/2011/sep/20/news/la-heb-diabetes-dementia-alzheimers-20110920

48 Chung, C., Pimentel, D., Jor'dan, A.J., Hao, Y., Milberg, W., Novak, V. (2015, July 8). Inflammation-associated declines in cerebral vasoreactivity and cognition in type 2 diabetes. Retrieved from http://www.neurology.org/content/85/5/450/. For an article written for the general public, see Park, A. (2015, July 8). How diabetes harms the brain. Retrieved from http://time.com/3948705/diabetes-harms-the-brain/

49 Holscher, C. (2018, June 15). New approach to Alzheimer's fight: Diabetes drugs. Retrieved from https://www.cnn.com/2018/06/15/health/alzheimers-insulin-study-partner/index.html

50 Researchers believe the sugar in breast milk—specifically lactose—feeds good bacteria in the infant gut. The sugar we eat as adults has the opposite effect by promoting the growth of bad bacteria in the gut.

51 For more on hidden sugars, see Bjarnadottir, A. (2017, June 3). The 56 most common names for sugar (some are tricky). Retrieved https://www.healthline.com/nutrition/56-different-names-for-sugar#section4

52 Imatome-Yun, N. (2015, April 16). How does fat affect insulin resistance and diabetes? Retrieved from https://www.forksoverknives.com/fat-insulin-resistance-blood-sugar/#gs.vx2nRh4

53 The value of coconut oil is highly debated because it is saturated fat (unhealthy), has medium-chain triglycerides (healthier than other forms of fat) and low levels of omega-6 fatty acids (healthy).

54 Harvard School of Public Health. Top food sources of saturated fat in the U.S. Retrieved from https://www.hsph.harvard.edu/nutritionsource/top-food-sources-of-saturated-fat-in-the-us/

55 Strawbridge, H. Artificial sweeteners: Sugar-free, but at what cost? Retrieved from https://www.health.harvard.edu/blog/artificial-sweeteners-sugar-free-but-at-what-cost-201207165030/

56 Oliveira, R. (2015 June). Why phytochemicals are important. Retrieved from https://ucdintegrativemedicine.com/2015/06/why-phytochemicals-are-important/#gs.Iv9YAtY

57 DeSilver, D. (2016, December 13). What's on your table? How America's diet has changed over the decades. Retrieved from http://www.pewresearch.org/fact-tank/2016/12/13/whats-on-your-table-how-americas-diet-has-changed-over-the-decades/

58 Micha, R, Wallace, S.K. & Mozaffarian, D. (2010, May 17). Red and processed meat consumption and risk of incident coronary heart disease, stroke, and diabetes mellitus: a systematic review and meta-analysis. Retrieved from https://www.ncbi.nlm.nih.gov/pubmed/20479151

59 Mozaffarian, D., Katan, M.B., Ascherio, A., Stampfer, M.J. & Willett, W.C. (2006, April 13). Trans fatty acids and cardiovascular disease. Retrieved from https://www.ncbi.nlm.nih.gov/pubmed/16611951

60 Villines, Z. (2017, November 30). What are the health benefits of beans? Healthline. https://www.medicalnewstoday.com/articles/320192.php. See also Say, J. (2015, March 9). 11 important health benefits of legumes—Reasons why you should consume more legumes daily. https://servingjoy.com/health-benefits-of-legumes/

62 Mattson, M.P. Energy intake, meal frequency, and health: a neurobiological perspective. Retrieved from http://www.ncbi.nlm.nih.gov/pubmed/16011467/; Matson, M.P. & Wan, R. (2005, March). Beneficial effects of intermittent fasting and caloric restriction on the cardiovascular and cerebrovascular systems. Retrieved from https://www.ncbi.nlm.nih.gov/pubmed/15741046

63 Gasior, M., Rogawski, M.A., & Hartman, A.L. (2006, September). Neuroprotective and disease modifying effects of the ketogenic diet. Behavioral Pharmacology: 17 (5-6), 431-439.

64 For more information, see Fan, S. (2013, October 1). The fat-fueled brain: unnatural or advantageous? Retrieved from https://blogs.scientificamerican.com/mind-guest-blog/the-fat-fueled-brain-unnatural-or-advantageous/

65 Harguth, A. (2017, January). These three classifications of food are based on Processed foods: What you should know. Retrieved https://mayoclinichealthsystem.org/hometown-health/speaking-of-health/processed-foods-what-you-should-know

66 Park, A. (2016, March 9). You won't believe how much processed food Americans eat. Retrieved from http://time.com/4252515/calories-processed-food/

67 If I can't pronounce an ingredient, is it bad? (2014, February). Retrieved from https://www.bestfoodfacts.org/cant_pronounce_ingredient/

68 Gunnars, K. (2017, June 4). Are nitrates and nitrites in foods harmful? Retrieved from https://www.healthline.com/nutrition/are-nitrates-and-nitrites-harmful#section6

69 Nitrates may be environmental trigger for Alzheimer's, diabetes and Parkinson's disease. (2009, July 6). Retrieved from https://www.sciencedaily.com/releases/2009/07/090705215239.htm

70 Butylated hydroxyanisole. (1991). Retrieved from https://ntp.niehs.nih.gov/ntp/roc/content/profiles/butylatedhydroxyanisole.pdf

71 I want to acknowledge immediately that a condition called hyponatremia, which results from too little salt, is also thought to increase the risk of dementia, but for Americans, this is an extremely rare condition—so low that I'm not going to further address it.

72 Faraco, G., Brea, D., Garcia-Bonilla, L., Wang, G., Racchumi, G., Chang, H., Buendia, I., Santisteban, M.M., Segarra, S.G., Koizumi, K., Sugiyama, Y., Murphy, M., Voss, H., Anrather, J., Iadecola, C. (2018, January 15). Dietary salt promotes neurovascular and cognitive dysfunction through gut initiated TH17 response. Retrieved from https://www.nature.com/articles/s41593-017-0059-z

73 Fiocco, A.J., Shatenstein, B., Ferland, G., Payette, H., Belleville, S., Kergoat, M., Morais, J.A., Greenwood, C.E. (2011, July). Sodium intake and physical activity impact cognitive maintenance in older adults: The NuAge study. Retrieved from this abstract: https://www.sciencedirect.com/science/article/pii/S0197458011002715?via%3Dihub

74 Abdoli, A. (2017, May). Hypothesis: High salt intake as an inflammation amplifier might be involved in the pathogenesis of neuropsychiatric disorders. Retrieved from https://www.researchgate.net/publication/316652319_Hypothesis_High_salt_intake_as_an_inflammation_amplifier_might_be_involved_in_the_pathogenesis_of_neuropsychiatric_disorders

75 Do I have to drink eight glasses of water per day? We asked five experts. (2018, April 12). The Conversation. https://theconversation.com/do-i-have-to-drink-eight-glasses-of-water-per-day-we-asked-five-experts-93025 (Be sure to "expand" each expert's comments to read what each said.)

76 Campaign for Dental Health. What do health experts say? Retrieved from http://ilikemyteeth.org/fluoridation/health-experts-on-fluoride/

77 Cornell, Paul. (2012, September). 50 reasons to oppose fluoridation. Retrieved from http://fluoridealert.org/articles/50-reasons/

78 Qtd. in Fact sheet: Bottled water and energy. (2007, December). Retrieved from https://www.banthebottle.net/bottled-water-facts/

79 Fishman, C. (2007, July). Message in a bottle. Retrieved from https://www.banthebottle.net/bottled-water-facts/

80 Toland, S. Why BPA-free plastic isn't necessarily safe. Retrieved from http://www.mensjournal.com/health-fitness/health/why-bpa-free-plastic-isnt-necessarily-safe-20140611

81 LaMotte, S. (2016, February). BPA-free plastic alternatives may not be as safe as you think. Retrieved from https://www.cnn.com/2016/02/01/health/bpa-free-alternatives-may-not-be-safe/index.html

82 Why are shower water contaminants dangerous to your health? (2018, May 2). Retrieved from https://epa-water.com/why-are-shower-water-contaminants-dangerous-to-your-health/

83 Hitti, M. (2006, February). Green tea may do wonders for the brain. Retrieved from https://www.webmd.com/food-recipes/news/20060217/green-tea-may-do-wonders-for-brain#1

84 Caffeine boosts enzyme that could protect against dementia. (2017, April 4). Retrieved from http://www.sleepreviewmag.com/2017/04/caffeine-boosts-enzyme-protect-dementia/

85 Sauer, A. (2017, January 4). 4 surprising benefits of coffee. Retrieved from http://www.alzheimers.net/2014-04-09/benefits-of-coffee/

86 Gunnars, K. (2017, June 4). Fruit juice is just as unhealthy as a sugary drink. Retrieved from https://www.healthline.com/nutrition/fruit-juice-is-just-as-bad-as-soda

87 Daily consumption of sodas, fruit juices and artificially sweetened sodas affect brain. (2017, April 20). Retrieved from https://www.bumc.bu.edu/busm/2017/04/20/daily-consumption-of-sodas-fruit-juices-and-artificially-sweetened-sodas-affect-brain/

88 Taylor, K. & Brodwin, E. (2016, November 16). There's a new big tobacco—and one industry is determined to silence its critics. Retrieved from http://www.businessinsider.com/big-soda-is-fighting-science-on-sugar-2015-11

89 For a balanced discussion of this topic, see McMillen, M. (2017, May 5). Is drinking diet soda a health risk? Retrieved from https://www.webmd.com/diet/news/20170505/diet-soda-health-risks

90 Ridley, N.J., Draper, B. & Withall, A. (2013, January). Alcohol-related dementia: An update of the evidence. Retrieved from https://www.ncbi.nlm.nih.gov/pmc/articles/PMC3580328

91 Inserm Press Office. (2018, February). Alcoholism and dementia risk. Retrieved from https://presse.inserm.fr/en/alcoholism-and-dementia-risk/30713/

92 American Addiction Centers. What are the links between alcohol and dementia? Retrieved from https://americanaddictioncenters.org/alcoholism-treatment/links-between-alcohol-and-dementia/

93 Montesinos, J., Alfonso-Loeches, S. & Guerri, C. (2016, November). Impact of the innate immune response in the actions of ethanol on the central nervous system. Retrieved from https://www.ncbi.nlm.nih.gov/pubmed/27650785

94 You can find many guides to drinking in moderation on the Internet. Here's one: HAMS Harm Reduction Network, Inc. (2015). Risk and alcohol drinking levels. Retrieved from http://hams.cc/limits/

95 Briggs, D. (2016 August 31). Worship: The weekend activity that can boost happiness, health throughout the week, studies find. Retrieved from http://www.huffingtonpost.com/david-briggs/worship-the-weekend-activ_b_11753778.html

96 This benefit is available to secular people as well—see the section on meditation.

97 Corsetino, E.A., Collins, N., Sachs-Ericsson, N., Blazer, D.G. (2009, December). Religious attendance reduces cognitive decline among older women with high levels of depressive symptoms. Journal of Gerontology: 64(12), 1283-1289.

98 Qtd. in UC Davis Health. (2015, November). Gratitude is good medicine. Retrieved from http://www.ucdmc.ucdavis.edu/welcome/features/2015-2016/11/20151125_gratitude.html. This website lists 12 ways that gratitude improves your health, including a decrease in neurodegeneration.

99 Emmons (see UC Davis note above) believes gratitude helps us to think about what we have rather than what we lack. You can decide who is right based on your own beliefs.

100 Gladding, R. (2016, Jul 4), The 'right' way to meditate: Practice—the mental gym—is what matters in meditation. Psychology Today. Retrieved from https://www.psychologytoday.com/us/blog/use-your-mind-change-your-brain/201607/the-right-way-meditate

101 See http://marc.ucla.edu/mpeg/03_Complete_Meditation_Instructions.mp3

102 EOC Institute. How meditation boosts 'BDNF'—keeps dementia Alzheimer's away. Retrieved from https://eocinstitute.org/meditation/bdnf-how-meditation-prevents-alzheimers-disease-dementia/

103 Giovanni. Scientific benefits of meditation: 76 things you might be missing out on. Retrieved from https://liveanddare.com/benefits-of-meditation/

104 For many more benefits, see Giovanni. Scientific benefits of meditation: 76 things you might be missing out on. Retrieved from https://liveanddare.com/benefits-of-meditation/

105 Learn more about Shinrin-Yoku at http://www.shinrin-yoku.org/shinrin-yoku.html

106 Jewish: Go to https://www.myjewishlearning.com/article/guided-meditation-for-the-high-holidays/; Islamic: http://www.islamicmeditation.com/main/audio-experience/; Christian: https://bitsofpositivity.com/free-guided-christian-meditations-for-teens-and-adults/ (you can also download the Abide app for a small fee). Many universities also offer their students free guided imagery downloads which you can use. Here are three: Dartmouth College: go to https://students.dartmouth.edu/wellness-center/wellness-mindfulness/relaxation-downloads; University of Iowa: go to https://www.counseling.iastate.edu/mind-body/mind-body-spa; CLA: go to https://www.uclahealth.org/marc/mindful-meditations

107 pEMFs differ from harmful EMFs based on exposure time, wavelength and frequency.

108 Your microbiome also includes your skin and a woman's vagina because these are accessible to the environment.

109 Hadhazy, A. (2010, February 12). Think twice: How the gut's 'second brain' influences mood and well-being. Retrieved from https://www.scientificamerican.com/article/gut-second-brain/

110 Galland, L. qtd. by Walravens, S.P. (2018, March 29). 10 signs you have a leaky gut—and how to heal it. Healthy Women. Retrieved from https://www.healthywomen.org/content/blog-entry/10-signs-you-have-leaky-gut%E2%80%94and-how-heal-it

111 Schroeder, B.O., Birchenough, G.M.H., Ståhlman, M., Arike, L., Johansson, M.E.V., Hansson, G.C., Bäckhed, F. (2018, January). Bifidobacteria or fiber protects against diet-induced microbiota-mediated colonic mucus deterioration. Retrieved from https://www.ncbi.nlm.nih.gov/pubmed/29276171

112 Sender, R., Fuchs, S. & Milo, R. (2016, August). Revised estimates for the number of human and bacteria cells in the body. Retrieved from http://journals.plos.org/plosbiology/article?id=10.1371/journal.pbio.1002533

113 Magnusson, K.R., Hauck, L., Jeffrey, B.M., Elias, V., Humphrey, A., Nath, R., Perrone, A., Bermudez, L. E. (2015, August). Relationships between diet-related changes in the gut microbiome and cognitive flexibility. Retrieved from https://www.sciencedirect.com/science/article/abs/pii/S0306452215004480

114 Sonnenburg, J.L. & Bäckhed, F. Diet-microbiota interactions as moderators of human metabolism. Retrieved from https://www.nature.com/articles/nature18846

115 Borchard, T. 10 ways to cultivate good gut bacteria and reduce depression. Retrieved from https://www.everydayhealth.com/columns/therese-borchard-sanity-break/ways-cultivate-good-gut-bacteria-reduce-depression/

116 Underwood, E. (2017, January 26). The polluted brain: Evidence builds that dirty air causes Alzheimer's, dementia. Retrieved from http://www.sciencemag.org/news/2017/01/brain-pollution-evidence-builds-dirty-air-causes-alzheimer-s-dementia

117 Air pollution. Retrieved from http://www.nationalgeographic.com/environment/global-warming/pollution/

118 Photo credit: Mnasiri7 Mansour Nasiri, licensed under the Creative Commons Attribution-Share Alike 3.0 Unreported license, retrieved from this website: https://commons.wikimedia.org/wiki/File:Baam_Tehran.gov

119 Your brain breathes too. (2014, January 29). Retrieved from http://knowingneurons.com/2014/01/29/your-brain-breathes-too/

120 Here's a list from NASA of houseplants that improve air quality: Knapp, J. (2016, January 29). 15 houseplants for improving indoor air quality. Retrieved from http://www.mnn.com/health/healthy-spaces/photos/15-houseplants-for-improving-indoor-air-quality/a-breath-of-fresh-air

121 World Health Organization. The impact of pesticides on health. Retrieved from http://www.who.int/mental_health/prevention/suicide/en/PesticidesHealth2.pdf

122 Pesticide-induced diseases: Alzheimer's disease. Retrieved from https://www.beyondpesticides.org/resources/pesticide-induced-diseases-database/alzheimers-disease

123 European Commission. Persistent organic pollutants (POPs). Retrieved from http://ec.europa.eu/environment/chemicals/international_conventions/index_en.htm

124 This list of fungicide alternatives comes from Genziuk, S. (2011, December 27). Natural fungicides for your garden. Retrieved from https://groundtoground.org/2011/12/27/natural-fungicides-for-your-garden/

125 Nelson, M. (2015, April 6). How to remove pesticides from your home in 8 simple steps. Retrieved from https://branchbasics.com/blog/2015/04/how-to-remove-pesticides/

126 For more on Integrated Pest Management, see: Snider, J. (2015, August 14). Integrated pest management: An inexpensive, safe, & sensible way to avoid pests. Retrieved from https://branchbasics.com/blog/2015/08/integrated-pest-management-an-inexpensive-safe-sensible-way-to-avoid-pests/

127 Roeder, A. Harmful, untested chemicals rife in personal care products. Harvard T.H. Chan School of Public Health. Retrieved from https://www.hsph.harvard.edu/news/features/harmful-chemicals-in-personal-care-products/

128 Meeker, J.D., Sathyanarayana, S., Swan, S.H. (2009). Phthalates and other additives in plastics: Human exposure and associated health outcomes, The Royal Society Philosophical Transactions B. Retrieved from https://www.ncbi.nlm.nih.gov/pmc/articles/PMC2873014/

129 Harmful chemicals in tobacco products. Retrieved from https://www.cancer.org/cancer/cancer-causes/tobacco-and-cancer/carcinogens-found-in-tobacco-products.html

130 Markesbery, W.R. The role of oxidative stress in Alzheimer disease. Retrieved from http://jamanetwork.com/journals/jamaneurology/fullarticle/775665

131 West, R., Beeri, M.S., Schmeidler, J., Hannigan, C.M., Angelo, G., Grossman, H.T., Rosendorff, C., Silverman, J.M. (2008, September). Better memory functioning associated with higher total and low-density lipoprotein cholesterol levels in very elderly subjects without the apolipoprotein e4 allele. Retrieved from https://www.ncbi.nlm.nih.gov/pubmed/18757771

132 Statin side effects: Weigh the benefits and risks. (2016, April 26). Retrieved from https://www.mayoclinic.org/diseases-conditions/high-blood-cholesterol/in-depth/statin-side-effects/art-20046013

133 Russel, P. (2016, April 20) Common meds linked to dementia. Retrieved from http://www.webmd.com/allergies/news/20160420/dementia-anticholinergic-medication#1

134 You can learn more about a medication check-up here: https://www.express-scripts.com/art/pdf/kap38Medications.pdf

135 Segell, M. (2011, November 3). Is dirty electricity making you sick? Retrieved from http://www.prevention.com/health/healthy-living/electromagnetic-fields-and-your-health

136 Tedeschi, C. (1997, February 3). Study finds electromagnetic fields may increase risk of Alzheimer's. Retrieved from https://news.usc.edu/12202/study-finds-electromagnetic-fields-may-increase-risk-of-Alzheimers/

137 Reducing electromagnetic fields. Retrieved from http://createyourhealthyhome.com/reducing-electromagnetic-fields/

138 Wu, M., Sass, J., Wetzler, A. (2010, April 30). Atrazine: Poisoning the well. Retrieved from https://www.nrdc.org/resources/atrazine-poisoning-well

139 United States Department of Agriculture, Animal and Plant Health Inspection Service, (Aug 17, 2015). USDA--APHIS--animal health--veterinary services--Center for Animal Health. Retrieved from https://www.aphis.usda.gov/aphis/ourfocus/animalhealth/sa_emerging_issues/ct_issues.

140 The FDA banned mercury in most cosmetics in 1974. It is still allowed at low levels in certain eye cosmetic products to prevent bacterial infections.

141 These fillings last longer but release low levels of mercury considered non-toxic by many authorities. You can ask your dentist for alternatives.

142 Simpkins, J. W. et al. (2009). The potential for estrogens in preventing Alzheimer's disease and vascular dementia. Therapeutic Advances in Neurological Disorders, 2(1), 31-49.

143 Effects of testosterone on your brain function. Retrieved from https://www.hgh.biz/blog/testosterone/effects-of-testosterone-on-your-brain-function/

144 Endocrine disrupting chemicals (EDCs). (2016, August 4). Retrieved from https://www.who.int/ceh/risks/cehemerging2/en

145 Gore, A.C., Crews, D., Doan, L., La Merrill, M., Patisaul, H., Zota, A. (2014, December) Introduction to endocrine disrupting chemicals (EDCs): A guide to public interest organizations and policy-makers. Retrieved from https://www.endocrine.org/-/media/endosociety/files/advocacy-and-outreach/important-documents/introduction-to-endocrine-disrupting-chemicals.pdf?la=en, p. 2

146 Diament, M. (2008, November). Friends make you smart. Retrieved from https://www.aarp.org/health/brain-health/info-11-2008/friends-are-good-for-your-brain.html

147 Here are two articles that might interest you: Granneman, J. (2017, August) You're not broken because you're an introvert. https://introvertdear.com/news/introvert-not-broken/ and Granneman, J. (2017, November) 17 signs that you have an introvert hangover. https://introvertdear.com/news/introvert-hangover-signs/

148 For more on forgiveness, see Brandt, A. (2016, May) How do you forgive even when it feels impossible. https://www.psychologytoday.com/us/blog/mindful-anger/201409/how-do-you-forgive-even-when-it-feels-impossible-part-1 and https://www.psychologytoday.com/us/blog/mindful-anger/201605/how-do-you-forgive-even-when-it-feels-impossible-part-2

149 Belluck, P. (2001, May 7). Nuns offer clues to Alzheimer's and aging. Retrieved from https://www.nytimes.com/2001/05/07/nuns-offer-clues-to-alzheimers-and-aging.html

150 Genova, L. What you can do to prevent Alzheimer'? Retrieved from https://www.ted.com/talks/lisa_genova_what_you_can_do_to_prevent_alzheimer_s/transcript?language=en

151 Effects of mental activity on health. Retrieved from https://www.myvmc.com/lifestyles/effects-of-mental-activity-on-health/

152 Effects of mental activity on health. Retrieved from https://www.myvmc.com/lifestyles/effects-of-mental-activity-on-health/

153 Qtd. in Adams, S. (2014, November 8) Proof that medication CAN grow your brain. Retrieved from http://www.dailymail.co.uk/health/article-2826953/Proof-meditation-grow-brain-just-eight-weeks-improve-learning-memory.html#ixzz4jhJ1f1NZ

154 How driving a taxi changes London cabbies' brains. Retrieved from https://www.wired.com/2011/12/london-taxi-driver-memory/

155 Maguire, E.A., Woollett, K. & Spiers, H.J. London taxi drivers and bus drivers: A structural MRI and neuropsychological analysis. Retrieved from https://www.ncbi.nlm.nih.gov/pubmed/17024677

156 Castro, J. (2011, May 24). The learning brain gets bigger—then smaller. Retrieved from https://www.scientificamerican.com/article/the-learning-brain-gets-bigger-then-smaller/

157 Barrett, L. F. (2016, December 31). How to become a superager. Retrieved from https://www.nytimes.com/2016/12/31/opinion/sunday/how-to-become-a-superager.html?_r=0

158 Barrett, L. f. (2016, December 31). How to become a superager. Retrieved from https://www.nytimes.com/2016/12/31/opinion/sunday/how-to-become-a-superager.html?_r=0

159 Unfortunately, it also follows that as people lose their ability to remember due to dementia, they also lose their ability to imagine. See An early silent burden of Alzheimer's: Losing imagination. (2015, September 28). http://www.afr.com/lifestyle/health/mens-health/an-early-silent-burden-of-alzheimers-losing-imagination-20150927-gjw4lk

160 Goodman, B. (2014, December 11). The promise and perils of brain training. Retrieved from http://www.webmd.com/news/breaking-news/brain-training/brain-training-promise

Acknowledgements

- **My father, Hassan,** who is my mentor and guide and who is battling this condition. His fight to win this battle inspired me to read, search and understand this condition. This book is a summary of my new knowledge and our journey. I love him so much.

- **All my teachers and mentors** who helped me to learn the art of medicine better and to **my patients**, who helped me understand medicine better.

- **Marilyn Kok,** my dear friend, who is gifted in converting complex information to very simple and bold communication for a specific audience. Her empathy and wisdom helped bring this book to life.

- **Amanda Van Rheeden**, a dear friend, who is passionate about health. She put the puzzle pieces together to make this book happen. I am sure she has a bright future in serving patients.

- **Jessica Michael**, a dear friend. As a caregiver herself, she understands the devastating nature of dementia. With her incredible talent, she produced illustrations that beautifully melded our information with visual representations.

- **Stephanie Cullen**, who provided the cover design and chapter art throughout the book.

- **David Cox**, who helped with editing and frameworking the book. His honest opinion guiding me in this journey has been invaluable.

- **Jackie Clayton, DNP, Libby Pasquariello, MSN/ED, RN, HN-BC, RYT, and Kathy Schanefelt, writer and editor**, who generously guided me, offering their point of view during this project. I have a great deal of gratitude for their efforts.

- **My family and friends** for their encouragement, listening, ideas and feedback.

- Last, but certainly not least, **my wife, Angela, and my kids** who donated countless hours of our quality time helping me write the book.

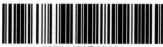

Made in the
USA
Lexington, KY